Live well; keep the faith utmost

Allen G Hulley MD
2012
Past Board member

# ACHIEVING
AND LIVING A HEALTHY
# LIFESTYLE
IN A WORLD OF STRESS

# ACHIEVING
## AND LIVING A HEALTHY
# LIFESTYLE
## IN A WORLD OF STRESS

**70 LESSONS FOR THOSE WANTING IMPROVED HEALTH
AND LOWER HEALTH CARE COSTS**

## ALLAN G. HEDBERG, Ph.D.
### FRESNO, CALIFORNIA

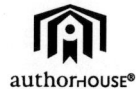

AuthorHouse™
1663 Liberty Drive
Bloomington, IN 47403
www.authorhouse.com
Phone: 1-800-839-8640


Order this book online at www.authorhouse.com.

© 2012 by Allan G. Hedberg, Ph.D. All rights reserved.

No part of this book may be reproduced, stored in a retrieval system, or transmitted by any means without the written permission of the author.


Published by AuthorHouse    04/04/2012

ISBN: 978-1-4685-5941-5 (sc)
ISBN: 978-1-4685-5940-8 (hc)
ISBN: 978-1-4685-5939-2 (e)

Library of Congress Control Number: 2012904877

Any people depicted in stock imagery provided by Thinkstock are models, and such images are being used for illustrative purposes only.
Certain stock imagery © Thinkstock.

This book is printed on acid-free paper.

Because of the dynamic nature of the Internet, any web addresses or links contained in this book may have changed since publication and may no longer be valid. The views expressed in this work are solely those of the author and do not necessarily reflect the views of the publisher, and the publisher hereby disclaims any responsibility for them.

Requests for information should be addressed to Allan G. Hedberg, 5100 N. Sixth, Suite 140, Fresno, CA 93710

Cover design: Benjamin C. Wolf and Lorens Lapinid
Interior design: Benjamin C. Wolf

# TABLE OF CONTENTS

## CHAPTER ONE

### CHOOSING A HEALTHY HEALTH CARE PROVIDER

The Marks of a Health Care Professional:
  A Personal Perspective ..............................................................1
The Healthy Lifestyle of a Health Care Professional ...................5
Negotiating With Your Health Care Provider ...............................9
Finding Help Through Psychotherapy .......................................11

## CHAPTER TWO

### PERSPECTIVES ON HEALTH AND HEALTH CARE

Women's Role Choices—Health and Work ...............................19
What Causes Poor Health? ........................................................21
The Stress of Divorce has Health Implications .........................23
The Health of the Homeless: Myths, Facts and Hope ...............25
The Dark Shadow Cast by Those Handicapped ......................29
Stress is Not a Stocking Stuffer .................................................31
Religious Faith and Health .........................................................33
Psychology Looks at Health Care .............................................37
Prescription Medication has a Dark Side Also .........................40
Learning From Success: The New Perspective
  of Positive Psychology ............................................................42
Is America the Leading Health Care Country in the World? .........44
Children and Stress: How to Help Your Children Cope ...............48

# CHAPTER THREE

## LIVING THE HEALTHY LIFE

The Importance of Good Communication.................................53
The Assertive Option of Communication ................................56
Smoke No More: Preparing for a Smokeless Life ....................60
Sleep Improves Health and Performance................................63
Real Men Cope Well.................................................................66
Loving Homes, Healthier Children.............................................77
Interpersonal Relationships Affect Health.................................79
In Search of the Healthy Family ...............................................82
Healthy Living Takes Time........................................................84
Happiness and Optimism: The Positive Alternative Lifestyle....86
Good Habits For Healthy Living.................................................93
Friends Make Good Medicine...................................................95
Controlling Arguments For the Sake of
   Your Relationships and Health .............................................97
Combating Loneliness is Combating Illness...........................100

# CHAPTER FOUR

## TURNING THE TABLE ON UNHEALTHY LIVING

Turning the Table on Stress...................................................105
Turning the Table on Depression............................................109
Myths About Depression......................................................... 111
Turning the Table on Burnout .................................................115
The Trauma Conundrum ........................................................119
The Pain of Discouragement: Is There a Way Out?...............125
The Eight R's of Anxiety Management ...................................128
Tempers Can Be Tempered...................................................131

Distinctives of the Type A Personality ......................................... 134
Coping Well With Pain, Illness and Disability ............................. 137

## CHAPTER FIVE

### COMMON HEALTH "PROBLEMS IN LIVING"

Liver Likes to be Cared for Too ................................................. 143
The Buddy System for Losing Weight ........................................ 148
The Bipolar Challenge ............................................................... 151
Migraine Headaches Strike Again .............................................. 157
Managing Gastroesophageal Reflux Disease (Gerd) ................. 160
Managing Chronic Pain .............................................................. 162
Insomnia: What is it and What Can We Do About it? ................. 168
Attention-Deficit Disorders and Hyperactivity ............................. 173
Hearing Loss Contributes to Depression and Dementia ............ 176
Depression Places Women at Risk for a Stroke ........................ 179
Coronary Heart Disease and Lifestyle ....................................... 181

## CHAPTER SIX

### AGING AS A CLASS ACT IN FINISHING WELL

What is this About Men Dying Before Women? ......................... 187
The Long Journey of Aging ........................................................ 191
Ten Key Factors to Consider When Choosing
   a Retirement Community ...................................................... 194
Retiring Seniors Take a Bow ..................................................... 198
Personal Legacy Letter .............................................................. 200
Memory Builders ........................................................................ 202
Brain Health Relates to Our Body Health .................................. 205
Coming to Terms with Loss and Grief ....................................... 208

# CHAPTER SEVEN

## CARETAKING AND ITS CHALLENGES

Words of Wisdom for Care Providers ............................................. 215
The Advantages and Benefits in Serving Older People ............. 217
Teenage Volunteers in a Skilled Nursing Home ........................ 221
Self Care for Care Providers ........................................................ 226
Making the Caretaking Experience Rewarding ......................... 229
Family Caregivers and Their Pressing Concerns ..................... 233

# CHAPTER EIGHT

## HEALTH CARE IN THE BUSINESS WORLD

The Benefits of an Employee Assistance Program (EAP)
    for the Worker and Employer ................................................ 237
Physician Stress and its Impact on Patient Care ....................... 240
Negotiating with Your Health Care Provider ............................. 244
When Depression Comes to the Work Place ............................ 248

**Epigraph**
Be Healthy ....................................................................................... 253

# ACKNOWLEDGEMENTS

In the production of any major work, numerous people play a significant role. They deserve acknowledgement:

. . . Bernice, my wife, for her constant help and assistance over 50 years of marriage.

. . . Gina, my secretary, for her extra efforts to see that deadlines and expectations are met.

. . . Oshea, my proofreader, for her sharp eyes and computer skills as the manuscript unfolded.

. . . Kathy, my typist, for her willingness to type a little later in the day to meet deadlines.

. . . Staff of Authorhouse, my publisher, for their readily available help and advice to bring the book to market in a timely manner.

# PREFACE

Every book comes about through some specific source of inspiration. This book is no exception. Two sources of inspiration have contributed to my writing and compilation of over 200 articles over the years of my professional practice as a clinical psychologist on a variety of subjects. Most of the articles were written in a desire to "give psychology away" to benefit my patients, audiences I addressed, and the general public.

First, during the forty years of my clinical practice, I have been fundamentally intrigued by the large body of research related to self-help. Indeed, hundreds of books have been written to help people help themselves in almost every problem area of life, such as toilet training, marital reconciliation, smoking cessation, bed wetting, fingernail biting, and being a first class parent, to name a few. Not only am I aware of this body of research, but have read many self-help books. I have also tried to follow the basic tenets of self-help in my professional and personal life. As I take care of myself, I am in a stronger position to care for others. Likewise, I encourage my patients to better care for themselves and improve their quality of health and relationships. To the readers of this book, I encourage you to do likewise.

The second inspiration came from my working as a professional therapist with a large number of patients such as Molly. Not long ago, Molly died at age 98.6 years of age. She was in relatively good health at the time of her death and essentially died of old age.

For fifty-five years prior to her death, Molly had not visited the office of a physician, and had no record of ever having taken a prescribed medication. She essentially cared for herself. She graduated from

*Allan G. Hedberg, Ph.D.*

high school, but was self-educated beyond her formal high school education. She maintained an active social life, and engaged in a regular habit of reading and self-education. She had an excellent support system. She ate moderately and her diet included an adequate supply of vegetables and fruits from her garden and backyard fruit trees. She loved an occasional donut and chocolate candy bar. She meticulously followed a sleep pattern of eight hours per night, and was often known to take a one-hour power nap each afternoon. Also, she was known to exercise by her daily walks until walking became an impossibility during her last five years of life. While her body grew frail, her mind remained sharp. Her attitude was always known to be positive.

Further, Molly was not one who consumed liquor, alcohol, tobacco, or other forms of self-medication. She did, however, use a general vitamin to supplement her healthy diet. Although unknown, it appears that she came from a very well honored and healthy genetic pool. Her family line all lived well and enjoyed a long life. They all finished well in their own time and in their own way.

While Molly has a story of her own, she really represents many people who engage in positive self-care and live a healthy life with little help from others, professionals or otherwise. Those like Molly are examples and models to all of us. They lead the way in healthy living by their own lifestyle choices and personal care.

Having now completed this book, I recommend it as I believe you will find encouragement to care for yourself and live a healthy life. I hope you will make corrections in some of your current health-related behavioral patterns and take direct personal responsibility for areas of your body and health that are out of whack and giving you "problems in living." Know that you can do better! You can live a healthy life as you move forward in your own journey of self-actualization.

Finally, as a reader of this book, I consider you a "second tier" patient of my clinical practice. I encourage you to take heed of the advice given in the various articles. They were written with you in mind. Your life can be enriched as were the lives of my patients over the years.

# Chapter One

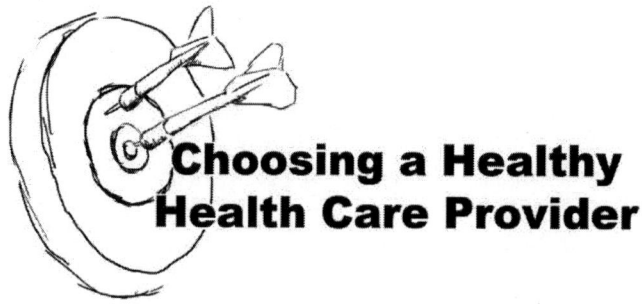

## Choosing a Healthy Health Care Provider

WITHOUT A SHEPHERD, SHEEP ARE NOT A FLOCK
*RUSSIAN PROVERB*

# THE MARKS OF A HEALTH CARE PROFESSIONAL: A PERSONAL PERSPECTIVE

Over the course of my professional training, I have been exposed to a wide variety of professionals from many different disciplines and personal opinions. Similarly, I was exposed to a host of different professionals through the influence of my parents, church, and the schools I attended. As a result of the opportunities afforded me through these contacts, I have come to formulate a view of a professional and have endeavored to pattern my professional life based on several "touchstones" of healthy professionalism. I share this model of professionalism; not as one who has attained, but as one who is always in the process of attaining.

If you are a person looking for a physician or therapist, I offer these guidelines for you to use as you ask various people for a referral or go about searching for the right person with whom to share your life and seek guidance for making necessary behavioral changes. Not every therapist is the same. Not all will be able to serve you well. The following guidelines should help make this choice easier and the person selected to be understanding, compassionate and helpful.

If you are a professional, join me in considering the marks of a professional as they pertain to you. May you find a model that you can use for shaping your own life and those for whom you hold a privileged responsibility. Consider the following marks of a health care professional:

*Allan G. Hedberg, Ph.D.*

## The Marks of a Health Care Professional

1. **A listening ear and sensitivity for what is being communicated, both verbally and non-verbally.** Before anyone can be in a position to assist and serve others, he/she or she must have developed the ability and the skills of acute listening. A good listener is one who is teachable, open, receptive and sensitive to the message and to the meaning of the message. The basic career of any professional begins with learning from others. Learning depends upon one's ability to attentively listen.
2. **A readiness and a knowledge of assessing a wide variety of ready resources.** Readiness means preparedness and availability. As a professional, he should have a sense of being prepared, available, and ready to respond to the needs of others while applying all of one's natural and learned resources, skills, talents, abilities, and experience. It involves being in a place of opportunity with a readiness to act as appropriate. Action means that one is ready, but also willing to step forward. This mark of a professional also means that one has access to a variety of resources beyond oneself that can be drawn upon as needed.
3. **The capacity for insightful compassion and understanding.** The role of the professional is to help, and this requires the ability to understand the need and respond in a caring and compassionate manner. The capacity for compassion generally is learned from the experiences that take place throughout the lifetime of the professional. Hurts, disappointments, achievements, tragedies, loss, and loneliness, to name a few, all coalesce in creating the capacity for compassion. Without it, a professional is incomplete.
4. **The attitude and humility of a servant.** We live in a profit-oriented society. We live in a world that emphasizes materialism and self-centeredness. True professionalism demands resistance to the temptation to put profit and self-interest ahead of service to others. A true servant does not act out of low self-esteem, but rather is one who has

already achieved a strong sense of self-confidence and self-regard. The actions of a servant do not reflect negatively upon the professional, but rather indicate the strength of the professional. The act of serving others is the giving of something valuable, not the attempt to satisfy one's own unfulfilled needs.

5. **A commitment to progressive continuing education and professional development.** We live in an age of information and the development of new ideas and new research findings. The increase of information is at a much greater rate today than ever before in history. A progressive professional is one who is committed to a personalized program of reading, personal study, attendance at educational and seminar events, and the integration of new information into one's personal life and professional practice. There is not only an awareness of new information and methods of approaching problems, but there is an updating of one's skills by which problems are approached and handled constructively and affirmatively. Professionalism demands the constant interchange of learning and applying.

6. **A commitment to self-care.** Professionals have a lot to juggle. This places stress on anyone, especially those responsible for the care of others. Too many place a low priority on self-care. In reality, self-care cannot be postponed. Research has shown that the lack of self-care leads to stress, distress and burnout. These factors can undermine one's competence and energy. It's an ethical priority and an imperative. It is a lifestyle, a life long habit.

In the process of attempting to articulate a model of professionalism or the general guidelines of a health care professional, it is easy to make it sound stiff, impersonal, and overly formal. While the guidelines might be written in objective terms, one must keep in mind that the professional, as a person, is human with his or her own frailties, sensitivities, values and preferred life style. The professional keeps in mind the fact that his or her own values and preferences must be understood and maintained in proper perspective and balance while serving others for the purpose of assisting them

*Allan G. Hedberg, Ph.D.*

reach their own goals and fulfill their own preferred directions in life. Further, it is important to realize that the professional appreciates the opportunity to be a positive influence in the life of others, but also appreciates what can be learned from others in the course of an ongoing professional relationship.

Learning is a two way street. Any benefit derived from professional services comes about as a result of an open, honest, and thorough analysis of a particular problem or issues of concern. No one has the corner on truth. We come to understand situations more clearly in the process of interaction and applying the principles of problem solving. Thus, the marks of a health care professional serve as overarching guidelines to every type of health care provider and their doctor/patient relationship.

# THE HEALTHY LIFESTYLE OF A HEALTH CARE PROFESSIONAL

When a person is looking for a physician, therapist or counselor, they look for certain characteristics that will likely generate confidence and a good therapeutic relationship. Often others are consulted in finding the right professional. The reputation of a physician or therapist is critical and often the determining factor for this critical decision. The following lifestyle characteristics of a health care professional are important for any potential patient or client to consider. All doctors are also encouraged to note these characteristics and heed them accordingly.

The lifestyle of a health care professional directly impacts the services and activities in which any professional engages. Lifestyle supports or hinders the services rendered. When there is a contradiction, a dissonance, between the lifestyle of the professional and the services rendered, a feeling of disappointment or lack of confidence towards that professional may result. Conversely, professional services can be enhanced and more effectively provided when the lifestyle of a professional is consistent with the services rendered and the principles or values espoused by the members of the general community being served.

Generally speaking, the lifestyle of a professional person needs to reflect dependability, energy and a broad fund of knowledge and experience. Also, the professional must have behavioral patterns based on articulated values, priorities and commitments. The actual skills and tools of a professional represent only a small portion of the ingredients for successful professional service. Who the professional is, and what he represents, speaks more loudly than what he does. People relate to the professional and seek out the services of the professional primarily because of the respect and confidence they have in that professional by observing how the professional lives and relates.

More specifically, the lifestyle of a health care professional needs to be developed so as to engender confidence, respect, trust and appreciation. A professional acknowledges that there are certain expectations which influence his acceptance by the community. There is little doubt that a professional person is expected to live a life above reproach and above that which is even tolerated for the general public.

The health care professional you select must be trusted, respected, and fully accepted before people will place their lives and their concerns in their hands for advice and direction. How then shall the professional live? What are the behavioral lifestyle traits and characteristics that engender respect, trust, and confidence? What is the lifestyle that goes beyond and supports the professional's technical expertise and competence? Consider the following:

## Lifestyle Characteristics of a Health Care Provider

1. **Is alert, energetic, responsive and sober in outlook.** Effective professional involvement requires alertness to the communication patterns going on and being specifically responsive to what is expressed and what is needed. This requires seriousness, conscientiousness, as well as sufficient energy to provide consistent service under stressful conditions. It is more than listening. People desire empathetic responsiveness to their expressed and unexpressed needs.
2. **Is of firm faith in himself and in the professional service rendered.** People have faith in another person to the degree to which they perceive that other person having faith in himself. Self-confidence engenders confidence from others. Confidence in the professional services one provides also encourages others to seek and utilize those services. It is

*Achieving and Living a Healthy Lifestyle in a World of Stress*

more than offering a professional service; it is believing in the value and quality of those services.

3. **Is faithful in serving others in the community.** Faithfulness is one of the most important trait we desire from those with whom we have relationships. Outcome or productivity is generally considered secondary to faithfulness and dependability. Good stewards of human resources are those who have been found to be faithful and just. Be available and reliable.

4. **Is known as a primary source of encouragement for all his contacts.** We are all attracted to those individuals who will provide us encouragement and emotional support. This is particularly true of those who feel lonely, insecure, and disparaged. There is an expectation of the professional to be above circumstances and to be a source of hope, belief, courage and future direction whenever needed.

5. **Is well trained and up-to-date in all areas of knowledge, facts and principles of problem solving.** Professionals are expected to be well-read and informed in their particular field, as well as on a variety of general topics. They are expected to be able to gather facts, think clearly, draw conclusions and suggest directions and guidelines from which others can benefit and bring order to their lives.

6. **Is unimpeachable in character and serves with integrity.** Confidence and credibility depend upon being perceived by others as living a lifestyle beyond reproach. Character is the reflection of basic commitments, beliefs and values. Character is learned from our daily life experiences and our response to those events. Integrity is the most basic ingredient of a relationship and serves to inspire others to follow and to learn from the professional interchange. The basis of any intimate relationship is respect for the integrity of each other.

The selection of a professional health care provider is one of the important decisions you will make in life. A mutual sense of trust is vital to a positive working relationship on behalf of your health and welfare. Your best interest must prevail in all decisions and medical

*Allan G. Hedberg, Ph.D.*

undertakings. Choose carefully and wisely. When choosing, check around and get the opinions of those that know the professional you are considering. While a perfect match may not be possible, it must be a good communicating and caring match.

# NEGOTIATING WITH YOUR HEALTH CARE PROVIDER

Would you be surprised to learn that only a small portion of patients pay 100% of the bill they receive from their health care provider for services rendered? This includes hospitals, clinics, labs, and specialists. It is not uncommon for a 10-30% discount to be arranged for lowering the final billing statement. Others commonly work out payment plans with a portion of the final billing being forgiven.

It is important to be aware of the fact that health care providers and medical facilities commonly have a rate schedule that is utilized differently for different consumers. Some are offered a lower rate, others pay higher. Fluctuation in the billing rate is not uncommon for most health care providers so patients might be encouraged to consider negotiating with their health care provider for an acceptable rate prior to the rendering of any particular service. Hence, negotiating may not only be a smart thing to do but it might be a prudent thing to do given your own financial circumstances and today's economy.

Remember, negotiations are not only permissible with physicians but also include physical therapists, psychologists, speech therapists, chiropractors, dentists, social workers, marriage and family counselors, and other types of health care providers. Remember that your health care provider must set fees and charge fees consistent with the patterns and ethics of their profession and in fairness to other patients. Negotiations can only go so far. Be realistic in your expectations.

Below are a few suggested negotiations that might be undertaken with your health care provider as you anticipate services being

*Allan G. Hedberg, Ph.D.*

rendered to you in the future. These might be negotiated each time a procedure is being undertaken, or as a general agreement that you establish with your health care provider for all services rendered in the future.

## Negotiating Considerations

1. With humility and respect, speak up assertively and ask for financial consideration.
2. Request a discount in fees upon your willingness to pay cash at the time services are rendered.
3. Ask if the treatment sessions can be sub-divided into smaller segments of time for a lower rate.
4. Ask if the treatment sessions can be spread out over an increased length of time from what was proposed so that payment is not burdensome in any given month.
5. Be honest and request special arrangements only if you really need it.
6. Request a payment plan over the course of 12 months but intend to have it paid off by then.
7. Ask for samples of medication and other medical supplies.
8. Ask for medications to be prescribed at the lowest cost, such as use of generics and equivalent medication that cost less than the brand name medication.
9. Ask to see a physician assistant, or other allied professional if the charges are less than those charged by the doctor.
10. Consider paying with your credit card to rack up mileage points for your next air flight.

# FINDING HELP THROUGH PSYCHOTHERAPY

Millions of Americans have found relief from depression and other emotional difficulties through therapy. Even so, some people find it hard to get started or stay in therapy. This brief question-and-answer guide provides some basic information to help individuals take advantage of outpatient psychotherapy.

## Why Do People Consider Using Therapy?

Therapy is a partnership between an individual and a professional who is licensed and trained to help people understand their feelings and assist them with changing their behavior. According to the National Institute of Mental Health, one-third of adults in the United States experience an emotional or substance abuse problem. Nearly 25% of the adult population suffers at some point from depression or anxiety.

People often consider therapy under the following circumstances:

- They feel an overwhelming and prolonged sense of sadness and helplessness, and they lack hope in their lives.
- Their emotional difficulties make it hard for them to function from day to day.
- Their actions are harmful to themselves or to others. For instance, they drink too much alcohol and become overly aggressive.
- They are troubled by emotional difficulties facing family members or close friends.
- They are facing a high stress event or trauma in their life.

*Allan G. Hedberg, Ph.D.*

## What Does Research Show About The Effectiveness Of Therapy?

According to a research summary from the Stanford University School of Medicine, therapy effectively decreases patients' depression and anxiety and related symptoms—such as pain, fatigue and nausea. Therapy has also been found to increase survival time for heart surgery and cancer patients, and it can have a positive effect on the body's immune system. Research increasingly supports the idea that emotional and physical health are very closely linked and that therapy can improve a person's overall health status.

There is convincing evidence that most people who have at least several sessions of therapy are far better off than untreated individuals with emotional difficulties. One major study showed that 50 percent of patients noticeably improved after eight sessions while 75% of individuals in therapy improved by the end of six months.

Research also shows that those with common mental health problems utilize less medical services and programs, such as ER visits, once they engage in a course of psychotherapy. They also make better use of the medication they have been prescribed.

Patient satisfaction is another significant component of effective therapy. A recent study by Avante Health found a 90% satisfaction level among a sample of patients served by their panel of therapists.

## How Do I Find A Qualified Therapist?

Selecting a therapist is a highly personal matter. A professional who works very well with one individual may not be a good choice for another person. There are several ways to connect with a qualified therapist:

- If you are planning to use your health insurance plan, call the insurance provider to obtain a list of therapists on their

panel. Also, get an authorization number for payments to be made.
- Talk to close family members and friends for their recommendations from the insurance company's panel, especially if they have had a good experience with therapy.
- Ask your pastor, teacher or primary care physician (or other health professional) for a referral from the therapist panel of your insurance carrier.

Ideally, you will end up with more than one lead. You may call and request the opportunity, either by phone or in person, to ask the therapist some questions. You might want to inquire about his or her licensure and level of training, approach to therapy, participation in insurance plans and fees. Such a discussion should help you sort through your options and choose someone with whom you believe you might interact well.

## What Makes A Good Therapist?

Research at the University of Wisconsin by Professor Wanpold has shown that a good therapist is known for the following characteristics:

- Has a sophisticated set of interpersonal skills.
- Build trust, belief and understanding from his patients.
- Develops a treatment plan but is flexible.
- Is reflective.
- Relies on the best research findings available.
- Monitors his patient's progress.
- Is influential, persuasive and convincing.
- Offers hope and realistic optimism.

## Once I Begin Therapy, How Can I Gain The Most From It?

There are many approaches to outpatient therapy and various formats in which it may occur—including individual, group and family therapy. Despite the variations, all therapy is a two-way process that works especially well when patients and their therapists communicate openly. Research has shown that the outcome of therapy is improved when the therapy is improved when the therapist and patient agree early about what the major problems are how therapy can help.

You and your therapist both have responsibilities in establishing and maintaining a good working relationship. Be clear with your therapist about your expectations and share any concerns that may arise. Therapy works best when you attend all scheduled sessions and give some forethought to what you want to discuss during each one.

Therapy isn't easy. But patients who are willing to work in close partnership with their therapist often find relief rom their emotional distress and begin to lead more productive and fulfilling lives.

## How Can I Evaluate Whether Therapy Is Working Well For Me?

As you begin therapy, you should establish clear goals with your therapist. Perhaps you want to overcome feelings of hopelessness associated with depression. Or maybe you would like to control a fear that disrupts your daily life. Keep in mind that certain problems require more time to resolve than others.

After a few sessions, it's a good sign if you feel the experience truly is a joint effort and that you and the therapist enjoy a good rapport. On the other hand, you should be open with your therapist if you find yourself feeling "stuck" or lacking direction once you've been in therapy awhile.

Patients often feel a wide range of emotions during psychotherapy. Some qualms about therapy that people may have, result from the difficulty of discussing painful and troubling experiences. When this happens, it can actually be a positive sign indicating that you are starting to explore your thoughts and behaviors.

After a brief series of therapy sessions, there should be evidence of fewer visits and referrals for medical care, ER visits, and general sickness. Physical health should show improvement also. This is called the "medical offset."

You should plan to devote some time in a session with your therapist periodically reviewing your progress. Although there are other considerations affecting the duration of therapy, success in reaching your primary goals should be a major factor in deciding when your therapy should end.

# Chapter Two

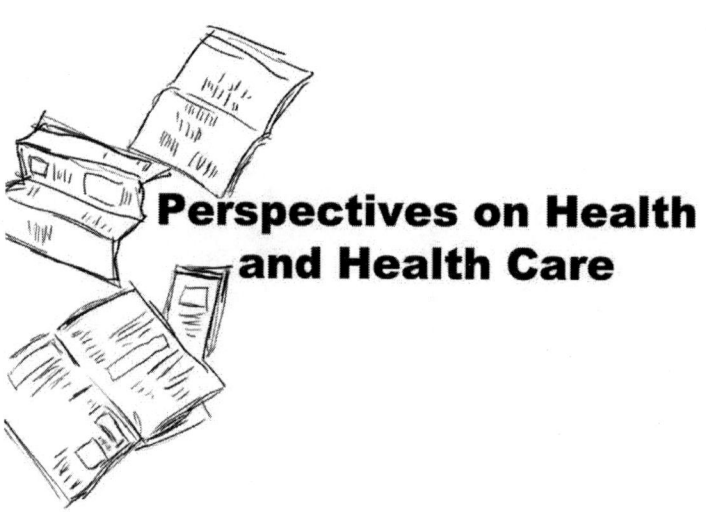

# Perspectives on Health and Health Care

HE WHO ENJOYS GOOD HEALTH IS RICH,
THOUGH HE KNOWS IT NOT
*ITALIAN PROVERB*

# WOMEN'S ROLE CHOICES—
# HEALTH AND WORK

Women become healthier as they are able to choose lifestyles they enjoy. So do their husbands who fully support those choices. Health care researchers expected to find that women's health would decline as they were exposed to the risks and stresses of the workplace. But an apparent narrowing of the differences in morbidity and mortality between men and women in recent years is more likely the result of improved health among men than declining health among women.

The researchers warn against drawing any definitive conclusions about these associations, and certainly about causation. The relationship between sex roles and health is complicated they noted, and the lag time between behavioral change and physical change is long. In general, the research findings indicate that working women tend to be happier and healthier, especially those working part time.

Louis Verbrugge, of the Institute of Gerontology at the University of Michigan, says women become healthier as they take on more responsibility. Employed married mothers are the healthiest, followed by employed married women with no children. Non-married women with no jobs or children are the unhealthiest, even after adjusting for the fact that many in this group are older widows. Marriage and family life seems to play a large role in a woman's health status. Part time work was an advantage.

There are exceptions. The trend does not hold, Dr. Verbrugge noted, for those with pre-schoolers or with three or more children, especially if they are unmarried and employed. And a Farmingham, Massachusetts, Heart Study found that clerical women had elevated coronary heart disease, but was thought to be associated with various social aspects of their job, especially poor relations with their bosses.

"Dissatisfaction with work is strongly associated with poor health for both men and women," Dr. Verbrugge said. "Women who are working by choice have better health, require less medical care, and use fewer medical drugs than do those women forced to work." This is also true of those who elect and are happy in a homemaker role, Dr. Verbrugge emphasized. The critical finding is that happiness matters in one's work, whether that is at home or at a paid job. Part time work yielded the most benefit for women in many areas of their life. Given the evidence that people with little social involvement have poor health, it may be wise to look at the stresses of social inactivity, work-related or otherwise.

Maintaining an active and healthy lifestyle which is satisfying to a woman is the key to good physical and psychological health. Whether this involves full-time homemaking, a career, or a combination of both, is not as important as how a woman may feel about her role choice. Even without limiting or restricting situations, choices are available which can help a woman feel better about herself and her world, such as changing jobs, retraining, returning to school, or volunteer work. The important thing to remember is that women have a role related choice, but it needs to be exercised.

# WHAT CAUSES POOR HEALTH?

Your emotions, attitudes, and behavior may be among the major determinants of your health according to an increasing number of experts from a variety of disciplines. "The premise that America's major health problems, namely heart disease, cancer, stroke, suicide, accidents and homicide are primarily caused by environmental factors and individual behavior and, therefore, cannot be solved solely by medical health services. This view has been endorsed by the U.S. Department of Health, Education and Welfare.

Several years ago, the American Psychological Association's Task Force on Health Research issued a report on the current status of and the dire need for research and consumer education on health related behaviors. The report identifies health as "one of the most crucial problems facing our nation," but notes that our methods of providing and financing health services are nearly exhausted. The health delivery system has not kept pace with the evolution over the years in fundamental preventive concepts relating to health and illness.

The Task Force report reviews the research on the relationship between social class and illness, hostility and hypertension, personality types and coronaries, and stress related depression and disease. Interest in the relationship between behavior and cancer is dramatically increasing. A number of psychologists have discovered a consistent description of the cancer patient as a rigid, authoritarian, inner directed and religious person, with ample conflict around sexual and hostile impulses, using excessive repression of affect and have poor emotional outlets. There is also data that indicates that cancer patients with a fast developing disease are more defensive and over-controlled than patients with slowly developing disease. There are other factors as well, to be sure.

Members of the Task Force found that "The amount of impact of research on the relationships between psychological factors and physical health are anemic," and they further indicated their intention to stimulate more interest in research on health behavior within the psychological community. The report concluded that "There is probably no specialty field within psychology which cannot contribute to the discovery of behavioral variables crucial to a full understanding of one's susceptibility." Physical areas open to psychological investigation range from health care practices and health care delivery systems to the management of acute and chronic illness. The psychology of medication benefit and pain management are others areas of ongoing study and understanding.

The new emphasis on improving health behavior requires greater individual responsibility for one's own health status and a reduced dependency on the health care system. The former Canadian Minister of Health and Welfare, Marc Lalonde, described this focus on individual behavior as a "cultural revolution," which will necessitate change in our eating, driving, drinking, smoking and exercise habits, as well as in our urban and job environments. "Health behavior" is a phrase Americans will be hearing frequently in the future, especially as health care is increasingly managed within a political context.

# THE STRESS OF DIVORCE HAS HEALTH IMPLICATIONS

There are a myriad of psychological interpersonal stressors that affect the quality of life, one's health and welfare, and even the duration of life itself. The death of a loved one, loneliness, conflict, trauma, and being rejected by a loved one are but a few strong examples of unwanted stress. On a scale of 1 to 100, divorce has the potential to disrupt biological processes that are important to a person's health and well-being. Not only do specific health problems develop, such as headaches, stomach aches, jaw pain, and fatigue, but so does there exist an increased risk for life-ending health problems.

Approximately two-million adults in the United States alone, end their marriage each year. When a couple divorces, one generally experiences more health impairment and lives a life of risk more than the other. Who fares well and who fares poorly is not entirely predictable. What we do know, is that one that fares poorly is at risk financially, medically, socially, vocationally, and spiritually.

Divorced individuals generally weather the storm of divorce better if they are forewarned, prepared, educated, and are capable of independent employment. They also do well if they possess strong self-reliant skills, have a strong social support network in place, and process the divorce proceedings in a civil, dignified and respectful manner. A recent survey of 32 separate research studies involving over 6-million people found that 160,000 deaths, and 750,000 divorces in eleven different countries revealed a significant increase in the risk for early death among those adults who were separated and/or divorced. By and large, older women and older adults fare better than men and younger adults, when death rates are taken into account following marital separation and divorce.

Further, the research found that adults who were divorced at the start of the research studies demonstrated a 23% increase in the probability of being dead from all causes when the sample was re-assessed at the end of the identified research study. That is, from the start of the divorce to a later point in time, a 23% increase in the probability of death was noted for those entering the status of being a separated or divorced individual. Men who were under the age of 65 years were at an elevated risk for early death relative to females and older participants. It is possible that men who by and large tend to isolate under stress and find it more difficult to reach out and initiate social network support, place themselves at greater risk as compared to women. Women generally are known to be more social and find access to social networks far better than men. The authors, Drs. David Sbarra, Rita Law, and Robert Porley, published the results of their study under the title of, "Divorce and Death: A Medi-Analysis and Research Agenda for Clinical, Social, and Health Psychology, 2011."

Should you be experiencing divorce or have recently entered into a divorce proceeding, be reminded of the high stress effects and the potential self defeating outcome that comes with it. Protect yourself and your marriage from the ill-effects of divorce, should that be your plight and circumstance.

In the face of divorce, do not isolate. Do not blame it all on yourself or all on your spouse. Do not drown your sorrows in alcohol or drugs. Do not work, exercise or read excessively as a way to run away from the negative effects of the divorce status. Rather, be forthright, assertive, socially and physically active, and engage in creative activities. Talk to others about your experiences. Talk to others about the quality of life after divorce.

# THE HEALTH OF THE HOMELESS: MYTHS, FACTS AND HOPE

Home, the place we take for granted. We have all reflected on the adages, "Home Is Where The Heart Is," "There Is No Place Like Home," and the popular song of years ago, "Home On The Range."

Home is viewed as a shelter, a place of domestic affections, a dwelling place, a retreat, and where we go to feel at ease and safe. It has been said, home is where they have to take you in when you show up.

For most of us, we experience daily the value and importance of a home. That includes many extended family members visiting or a period of quietness and rest in the safety of our home. Unfortunately, for some, there is no home. Such people are known today as the homeless. They are all around us. We see evidence of the homeless population and the factors that have encouraged it. On any given night, about 5,000 people in Toronto, 900 people in Ottawa and 2,700 people in Vancouver are homeless. Over the course of a year, and estimated 150,000 to 300,000 Canadians will experience homelessness.

Recent surveys estimate that .06% of the population in a major city such as Las Vegas is homeless, including adults and youth.

## Homeless and Health

People who are "vulnerably housed"—meaning they live in unsafe, unstable or unaffordable housing—had equally poor, and in some cases worse, health.

*Allan G. Hedberg, Ph.D.*

The St. Michael's Hospital issue of *International Journal of Public Health* reported from a study that over 50% of the Canadian homeless have mental health problems; 85% have chronic health conditions.

The underlying cause for these health issues is poverty, said Dr. Stephen Hwang, the principal investigator of the study and a physician-researcher at the hospital's Centre for Research on Inner City Health.

Participants in the survey reported having at least one chronic health condition, such as diabetes and heart disease, and more than 50% reported being diagnosed with a mental health problem. Previous research has found that homeless people have much poorer health than other members of society.

The 2007 Street Health Report, a survey of the health status and needs of homeless people in downtown Toronto, found that while 61% of the general population reported that they were in excellent or very good health, only 29% of homeless people felt they were in excellent or in very good health.

While 40% of homeless people said they were in fair or poor health, only 9% of the general population responded that they were experiencing fair to poor health status.

## Who Are the Homeless?

**Myth:** The homeless are homeless by choice.
**Fact:** Contrary to the popular stereotype, almost one in five of the homeless population is working. Further, the major victims of homelessness are children. Very few people choose to be homeless. Most are forced into homelessness by circumstances, such as, losing work, lack of affordable housing and the absence of a supportive family or a social network.

**Myth:** Once homeless, always homeless.

**Fact:** Most homeless people are homeless for brief periods of time. It is estimated that 4-5 times the permanent homeless people are those who experienced periodic or seasonal homelessness.

**Myth:** The homeless population is made up almost entirely of single adults.
**Fact:** According to the U.S. Conference of Mayors, families and children make up the fastest growing segment of the homeless population. The Department of Housing and Urban Development estimated that families with children comprise 40% of the homeless population. In some cities, such as New York, Philadelphia and Portland, families comprise over half of the homeless populations. Further, the Department of Health and Human Services estimated that there were more than a million runaway and homeless youth, ages 10-17.

**Myth:** The vast majority of the homeless are mentally ill.
**Fact:** The National Institute of Mental Health estimates that approximately 30% of homeless individuals are mentally ill, although the percentage varies from area to area.

## Why be Concerned?

If current trends continue, by the year 2025, multi-millions of American children will have spent at least part of their childhood without a home. These children will carry the physical, educational and emotional scars of a childhood marked by cold, hunger, sporadic schooling, and the impoverished environment of a shelter.

A number of studies have documented the serious emotional consequences of homelessness on children. For example, one study of 156 homeless children in Boston found that a majority of these children seriously thought about killing themselves. Other studies show how the chaotic environments of the shelters and welfare hotels have severe and lasting effects on normal maturation and development. These children have reduced potential for a productive and independent adult existence. Dr. Hwang says, "We need to treat both problems."

## Can We Help the Homeless?

The most economically and socially vulnerable members of society are at greatest risk for becoming homeless. Healthy communities help by designing and providing much needed supportive services, such as substance abuse treatment, day care and health clinics. Such services may be necessary to help the homeless toward an independent lifestyle—or prevent families and individuals from becoming homeless in the first place. Most helpful are the entrepreneurial efforts in a community designed to provide employment training, skill development, income production, remedial education and learning the English language.

Caring individuals play a major role by contributing food, clothing, furniture and other items to the agencies and organizations within the community serving the homeless. Local agencies are most appreciative of any contribution that would help them continue their task in serving a very needy segment of the community on our behalf.

However, there are two options. We are reminded and should not forget the guidance offered in the adage, "Give a man a fish and he'll eat for a day, but teach him how to fish and he'll eat for a lifetime." While a healthy and compassionate community does both, the focus is best placed on being a teaching community. Teaching communities are win-win communities.

# THE DARK SHADOW CAST BY THOSE HANDICAPPED

We have all met or come into contact with a person who was different from our perception of normal. Perhaps this person spoke with a peculiar accent, or perhaps was blind, deaf or learning disabled.

We live in a society where stigma is rampant. According to Erving Goffman, the term "stigma" refers to a deeply discrediting trait. He states that it may also be called a failing, a shortcoming, or a handicap. People often develop assumptions about what characteristics others should posses. We tend to set standards as to how others should appear, behave, or think. We, who believe ourselves to be normal, develop the stereotypes of normal behavior. As a result, people who do not measure up to these standards become failures. According to Goffman, people who fall short become reduced in our minds from a whole and normal person. They are tainted, and discounted. Criminals, ethnic Americans, and handicapped individuals have often been stigmatized as outsiders and seen as less than fully human. Communities can easily become "communities of rejection."

The physically disabled are definitely stigmatized. Physical disabilities are clearly looked down upon. We tend to experience awkwardness, strain and inhibition when interacting with someone who is disabled, because they are "different." We have difficulty admitting that our attitudes toward the disabled are typically less favorable than our attitudes toward the non-disabled. Persons with disabilities may not measure up to our standards because we see ourselves and the world as better and "non-disabled."

*Allan G. Hedberg, Ph.D.*

In order to eliminate this interpersonal prejudice within ourselves, we must all realize that we all have some degree of disability, whether it is a mental, physical, emotional, or a learning impairment. Having the ability to understand our own limitations, accept them, and feel good about ourselves is essential for healthy daily living. Understanding our own disabling condition and the handicapping factors is no easy task. First, there is the obstacle of understanding. When a person has to adjust to a new or unusual set of limitations, a period of uncertainty naturally results. It is important to receive information about the particular disability. This can be done through reading and interacting with other people who have the same or similar disabilities. Learning about the experiences and thoughts of other disabled individuals is very useful in developing a healthy attitude about one's own unique disability.

Once we understand our own disabling condition, the real battle begins. Reconciling our personal needs with the handicapping barriers placed upon us by society and the environment is generally more difficult than a physical impairment itself. The challenge is for us to communicate with one another about our needs and frustrations without feeling stigmatized. Consistent with the Golden Rule, we must learn to treat each person in the way we want to be treated. Clearly, we all want the best for our lives, whether we be handicapped or not. We all want growth so that we can become the best we can be.

# STRESS IS NOT A STOCKING STUFFER

The Christmas and New Year holidays are to be a time of joy, sharing, contentment and connecting with our loved ones. Unfortunately, the storybook holidays just do not come true for many of us. For some of us, the holiday blues and depression can be a sad reality. For some it is a time of meaningful celebration.

To prevent depression over the holidays, it is important to take particular steps to be around others who care and provide positive and supportive companionship. Consider the following stress reducing gifts brought to all of us by the famous eight reindeers:

*Reindeer 1.* **Stress proof yourself** by lightening your load and planning for times of fun in your schedule. Do not try to have a picture book perfection holiday schedule and experience. Be realistic.

*Reindeer 2.* **Limit spending** by sticking with a realistic budget for gifts, food and travel. Do not over-use credit cards. Moderation is the word.

*Reindeer 3.* **Plan family time** by scheduling events such as a drive down Christmas Tree Lane, watching a special television Christmas concert or program, taking a family hike together or creating a new and unusual holiday tradition for the family.

*Reindeer 4.* **Give "non-monetary" gifts** such as promising to do a favor for someone, doing chores for someone, or some other random gifts of kindness.

*Reindeer 5.* **Create a meaningful gift attitude** and not give gifts to impress but give only to those who really need or will appreciate your gift. Cut your gift list to a reasonable number of names. You don't have to give to all or give a bigger gift than you received last year.

*Reindeer 6.* **Be a smart shopper** by finding something on sale and buying many of them to give to those on your list. Also, try to shop alone whenever possible so you have a sense of peace. Farm the kids out so you can shop peacefully.

*Reindeer 7.* **Enjoy the true meaning of the holidays** by expressing your love and gratitude in many ways other than gift giving. Express your feelings in cards and personal notes to those for whom you are grateful.

*Reindeer 8.* **Read the Christmas Story** as recorded in the second chapter of Luke of the Bible. Read it in different translations of the Bible. Talk about it with others until it becomes a meaningful story to you and your family.

An abundant life, a peaceful life, and a victorious life are possible even at times of stress such as Christmas and the New Year. Enjoy the Season with your family, friends and associates without being disabled by stress.

# RELIGIOUS FAITH AND HEALTH

It is not uncommon to hear people say that they truly believe God carried them through a particular crisis in their life, such as a divorce, job loss, a major health reversal, or a financial setback. Many doctors acknowledge the power of faith at work in the lives of their patients. Church attendance generally increases for a few months following a national disaster, such as 9/11. According to a survey published by Trinity College in Harvard, Connecticut, 70% of Americans believe in God and that he has something to do with the events of the world. Three out of four Americans engage in prayer regularly. Prayer is generally considered beneficial to cognitive functioning, stress relief, improved emotional states, life and death situations, and decision making, to name a few areas of positive impact.

## Religion and Health

Michael E. McCullough of the University of Miami is probably recognized as one of the most prolific researchers on the relationship between religion and health. He has written dozens of reports on this subject. A sampling of his research findings include the following observations:

1. Religious people of all faiths do much better in school, live longer, have more satisfying marriages, and are generally happier than those who are similarly situated but identify as non-believers.
2. In a major study consisting of over 125,000 people, those that were religious were 25% more likely than the non-religious

individuals to live longer than the norm for their demographic group.
3. In the area of addiction, the cessation of smoking is better among religious people. Similarly, church attendance helps an individual come to terms with alcohol addiction more than Alcoholics Anonymous.
4. Health and prosperity indicators are higher among religious people. This seems to be related to the fact that they have better self-control.
5. Prayer has been generally found to have powerful affects on the body. Scientists have found that images of the brain at the time of prayer resemble that of a person interacting with someone they love.
6. People who attended religious services more than once a week over the course of a year were 24% less likely than non-church attenders to abuse alcohol.
7. A survey of 64 different studies about religion and health found a pattern between regular worship service attendance and a reduction in health-related problems, such as hypertension and heart attacks. Religious people were particularly good at handling physical pain.

## Prayer and Health

Research at the Brandeis University on religion and health focused on the effects of intercessory prayer for sick people. They found conflicting results suggesting that prayer benefits some while others it did not.

Another study on prayer as religious coping was conducted at Regent University. It was found that prayer, defined as people's vehicle for communicating with God, was more influential and stress reducing than the usual therapeutic procedure of journaling. Prayer offered additional stress relief even beyond religious thoughts or meditations. Other research has found that effective prayer is a "time of prayer" (i.e., 20 minutes), not just a fleeting moment of prayer.

In another series of research studies conducted at the University of Montgomery the researchers found that patients undergoing hospice benefited from their faith. They experienced increased comfort by their relationship with God, by believing in the hope of life after death, and through the reassurance of a cosmic order, design and purpose for life and death.

Another study conducted at Brandeis University found that prayer among patients with serious medical problems is generally raised by a family member rather than their doctors. Coming out of all the research findings was the recommendation that medical education needs to include time for the consideration of prayer as part of medical practice and relationships with patients of all faiths. Some doctors were found to participate in religious rituals such as baptism at bedside while others preferred to remain distant from the religious exercise taking place at bedside. Some doctors are afraid to become involved in a religious ritual or respond to such requests as they do not want to appear to have more power to cure the patient than actually is the case.

Generally speaking, physicians desire to be respectful of a family's prayer time even if they did not want to participate or share in the family's religious or spiritual beliefs and practices.

## Religion and Depression

Further, research conducted at Colombia University consistently found that adult women with a history of lifetime depression indicated an inverse association between religiosity and symptoms of depression. Further, they found over ten years a long-term protective effect against depression for those who placed a high importance on religion and their spirituality. Growing out of this body of research has been a spiritually integrated form of psychotherapy for patients with depression. It has been helpful for some patients.

At the Rush University Medical Center in Chicago a fairly extensive study of 136 adults diagnosed with Major Depression or Bipolar

*Allan G. Hedberg, Ph.D.*

Disorder found that those with strong belief and concern for God were more likely to experience improvement in their state of depression over time. The study concluded by indicating that treating doctors need to be aware of the role of faith in their patient's life when they develop a care plan and begin to treat the depressed person.

In summary, much ongoing research is taking place at many universities on all aspects of faith and health. So far, faith has been found to be a positive influence on the lives and healing process of patients with a variety of health issues.

# PSYCHOLOGY LOOKS AT HEALTH CARE

## We All Benefit From Psychological Research

Psychology plays a major role in solving individual, social, industrial, educational and health care problems in advancing the quality of our lives. Few among us understand psychology's contribution to health care particularly. Most think of psychology only as it relates to mental health. Mental health is an important area for psychological research and practice, but psychology is much more than that. Psychology is the science of how we behave—and why we behave as we do in all kinds of settings and under a variety of circumstances.

As a science, psychology encompasses research on behavior at very different levels. Areas include the reaction of the human eye to different colors and intensities of light, the study of how individuals form opinions and attitudes, our understanding of the developmental stages in children, and the behavior patterns that influences our health and welfare, for example.

Psychological research has produced important results that help us to be more productive at work, more attentive in school, travel more safely, and live healthier lives. Often these advances are less obvious to consumers than the products and technology of other fields of science. However, the benefits of psychological research are just as real as those of complex computers, and just as significant as improvements in medical care. The historical contributions of psychological research underscore the solid foundation of basic and applied research.

*Allan G. Hedberg, Ph.D.*

## Applied Psychological Research

The following examples illustrate some of the benefits to society of applied psychological research. There are many other areas of study and benefit, but the sample below will give an idea of psychology's contributions to society.

1. Basic research on attitude change and persuasion has led to the improvement of American's health status and the savings of millions of dollars. Convincing people to maintain programs of preventive health care has been made easier through behavioral research. For instance, research psychologists have learned how to motivate patients with high blood pressure, to change their diets and food selection, and continue compliance in taking their medication. This has resulted in greatly improved health for millions of Americans, as well as tremendous savings in health care costs.
2. Many body functions, like blood flow, hand moisture, and heartbeat, are usually considered automatic. Through the use of biofeedback technology, accurate information about one's automatic bodily functioning is provided to an individual. Psychologists have shown that this information will allow the conscious control of these and other automatic functions. This is known as Bio-feedback training and can improve one's overall health.

Biofeedback can help people fight many physical disorders such as migraine headaches, low back pain, and nausea from cancer chemotherapy. Biofeedback is considered by many to be the treatment of choice for these and other medical disorders, saving enormous costs over alternative medical treatments and avoiding complications of long-term drug use. For example, the use of biofeedback has been shown to reduce the number of severe seizures in persons with epilepsy, and has even worked when drug treatments have not. The field of biofeedback has grown to become a major treatment alternative for many medical and psychological disorders.

3. Because of the psychological studies of environmental design, a major metropolitan hospital in New York City better understands how the physical environment of the hospital affects patients, staff, and visitors. These environmental psychological studies were designed to discover how a hospital can reduce stress for both employees and patients and also promote healing. Results from these studies are being used in a continuing program of design changes for hospital facilities and their operation. This work has grown out of basic psychological research on the effects of the environment on behavior and emotions.
4. Psychologists have also been studying the effects of noise, heat, and repetitive tasks on the ability of workers to remain alert and safe. Safer and more productive workplaces have resulted from these studies.

## Summary

Our world is changing more profoundly than most of us realize. It is clear that critical resources will continue to be in limited supply. The most important of these is our human resources—the trained minds dedicated to solving the increasingly complex problems of humankind. Although we will depend on science and technology to solve many of our problems, we cannot depend solely on "hardware" solutions. Many of our continuing world problems must be solved through behavioral and psychological research and application. The future of all nations of the world rests on a better understanding of human thinking, human commitment, and human ingenuity. The support of behavioral science research is a sound investment in our nation's future.

# PRESCRIPTION MEDICATION HAS A DARK SIDE ALSO

The mere mention of drug addiction generally conjures up images of ill-kempt, uneducated, and unemployed users of heroin and crack cocaine. To be sure, this is one image of the dark side of a community. On the other hand, there is a growing number of individuals around the world that are dependent on legal drugs, prescribed by their physicians, with a grip as unforgiving as that of their illegal counterparts. This problem does not just take place on the street corner, empty apartment, or back alley of a community, but in the sterilized offices of our medical doctors. It has become a problem that cannot be ignored. Unfortunately, the depth of prescription medication addiction, especially related to pain killers and tranquilizers, remains low on the agenda of the medical community, pharmaceutical community, and the governmental community.

Opioid pain killers are being dispensed through the use of a prescription at five times the rate they were twenty years ago. A review by Great Britain's National Treatment Agency for Substance Abuse found a six-fold increase in the prescribing of opioid analgesics by general practitioners from 228-million items in 1991 to 1.38 billion items in 2009. Further, deaths by the use of codeine has doubled between 2005 and 2009 alone. It is estimated that 1.5 million people could be hooked on such medication in Great Britain alone. There are many more who are unaware they have a problem and, unfortunately, there is little support or help for those that do. Medication addiction requires more than a piece meal approach, but a comprehensive strategy to control such medication accessibility and treatment for those addicted. Of course, preventative information and approaches are also found wanting. With the growing battery of medications to combat chronic pain, chronic anxiety, and other emotional distresses, those suffering from such disorders are keen to make use of these medications, especially the newer ones coming on the market. The miracle cure to solve an emotional or physical area of distress is still the obsession among those suffering from chronic disorders. The increasing use of such medication represents a "disaster in the making."

Patient demand upon their personal and family physician is the driving force upon drug companies to market such medication. Marketing strategies and techniques are increasingly being aimed at potential users, the chronic pain patient, as compared to the direct appeal to the medical community itself. It is well-recognized that throughout America, the U.K., and across Europe the population is aging. This translates into an anticipated increase in the incidents of chronic pain-related conditions such as arthritis and fibromyalgia. Chronic pain, anxiety and depression are directly involved in such medical conditions. A call for more and more medication is unprecedented.

Chronic pain and mental anguish caused by injury or chronic disease has been poorly treated in the past. Physicians acknowledge the growing use of powerful pain killers as a sign of a more compassionate society that is prepared to comfort those in need. However, there is a risk. As doses rise and dependency grows, dangers outweigh the potential benefits. There is a growing battery of drugs to combat anxiety and chronic pain, but a balance must be struck so that the benefits continue to outweigh the risks.

Dr. Kathy Stannard, the author of Opioids in Chronic Pain said, "There has been a huge increase in prescribing the opioid pain killers and they are being overused. Patients keep going back to their doctors complaining of pain and the doctors don't know what to do, so they increase the dosage." With other conditions, if the drug isn't working, doctors stop it and try something else. But it doesn't seem to be a common medical practice for doctors to say, "If this pain killer isn't working, we should stop it."

# LEARNING FROM SUCCESS: THE NEW PERSPECTIVE OF POSITIVE PSYCHOLOGY

Over the past 100 years, psychology and the behavioral sciences have studied people whose lives were in distress and where a breakdown in performance occurred. Psychology has based its theories and its methods of therapy on the data collected from this "particular sick clinical population." More recently, a quiet revolution has been taking place. We have learned that social and personal problems do not necessarily improve when we apply our strategies based upon the experiences of individuals and organizations that have failed or shown some level of disability. That approach has not necessarily turned around the divorce rate, the amount of alcoholism and drug abuse in our society, or the occurrence of stress related health disorders. A new approach has been needed and is now emerging.

More recently, psychology has started to look in a new direction focusing on wellness for greater understanding and answers. As a result, a considerable amount of time is being devoted to the study of people whose lives are well functioning and who bring honor to their families, communities, and their companies. In-depth studies are being undertaken involving people who are succeeding vocationally, romantically, and physically. Exciting and positive findings are beginning to appear as we research successful and healthy individuals, couples, children and corporations.

A few examples of this new research development are as follows: 1) Identifying those individuals that thrive, even in stressful situations. 2) Identifying the body's "nutritional requirements" for healthy behavioral responses under adversity. 3) Identifying those vital characteristics of business that succeed and grow. 4) Identifying the traits of strong and successful families and marriages.

5) Identifying the factors that are associated with living to 100 years of age. 6) Identifying the factors that lead one person to rely heavily on physicians and have frequent appointments and another person to live years in good health and not see a physician for 50 or more years.

It was the famous scientist, Louis Pasteur, who developed the germ theory as the basis for causing disease. On his deathbed, his theory was changed. He stated, ". . . the germ is nothing, the host is everything . . ." This major refocus in thinking represents major redirection in the field of medicine and behavioral science. The disease is not just a germ, but the body's inability to fight germs, foreign invaders, body parasites and other similar attackers. From this change in thinking and research, we have come to learn that the immune system is the key for promoting and maintaining health. We must protect it and respect it.

Likewise, we are becoming increasingly aware of the significant role played by the environment in which an individual lives—the work, home, school, and social environment. It is the dynamic interaction that takes place between an individual and his or her environment that determines effective living. Environmental change often results in behavior and performance change in the people affected by that environment.

In summary, psychology and other fields of understanding have advanced our knowledge of human behavior up to now with a strong focus on what went wrong. Already, we are experiencing a significant surge in our data base an understanding of human behavior by our intentional refocus on wellness and positive behaviors and outcome. As we look forward, it is anticipated that many new relationships and understandings will emerge. We especially look for new developments in healthcare. We desire to learn more of how to care for oneself, reduce health care costs, how to live a healthy lifestyle, and how to foster healthy communities. Self defeating behavior must and will be replaced by self enhancing behavior patterns. We are well on the way towards making this a reality.

# IS AMERICA THE LEADING HEALTH CARE COUNTRY IN THE WORLD?

It is a common belief that America is the country that leads the world in health care. Recent studies bring this into question. In 2008, Dr. Barbara Starfield published in *The Journal of the American Medical Association,* the results of a public health study in which the United States health care system was compared to 12 other industrialized countries. Included in this study were Japan, Sweden, Canada, France, Australia, Spain, Finland, The Netherlands, The United Kingdom, Denmark, Belgium, and Germany. The results of her study indicate that the U.S. ranked at or near the bottom in several significant health care indicators when compared with these 12 countries. The results on several indicators are noted below:

**HOW U.S. RANKS ON SEVERAL SIGNIFICANT HEALTH CARE INDICATORS:**

- 13th (last) for low-birth-weight percentages
- 13th for neonatal mortality and infant mortality overall
- 11th for postneonatal mortality
- 13th for years of potential life lost (excluding external causes)
- 12th for life expectancy at 1 year for males, 11th for females
- 12th for life expectancy at 15 years for males, 10th for females

Perhaps more shocking was the finding that iatrogenic damages were the third leading cause of death in the United States after heart disease and cancer. An iatrogenic damage is defined as a state of ill health or adverse effects resulting from a specific medical place or treatment. That is, the treatment procedure or facility itself caused some type of unintended injury, damage or was the cause of death. The finding indicates in brief that doctors and hospitals that provide certain treatments are more responsible for deaths and ill-effects on a patient than respiratory diseases, accidents, diabetes, pneumonia or cerebral-vascular disease.

The combined adverse effects of errors that occur because of iatrogenic damages resulting in deaths include the items as outlined below:

---

**COMBINED ERRORS AND ADVERSE EFFECTS OF IATROGENIC DAMAGES:**

- 12,000 deaths/year from unnecessary surgery
- 7,000 deaths/year from medication errors in hospitals
- 20,000 deaths/year from other errors in hospitals
- 80,000 deaths/year from nosocomial infections in hospitals
- 106,000 deaths a year from nonerror, adverse effects of medications

---

As can be noted, infections acquired in a hospital, and errors and adverse effects of medication appear to be the leading causes of iatrogenic deaths. The total results in more than 225,000 deaths per year from iatrogenic causes. That number does not include adverse effects associated with disability and discomfort, but only reports of actual deaths. Other reports by the Institute of Medicine indicate deaths as high as 284,000 annually. Further, the World Health Organization issued a report in the year 2000 noting that the U.S. ranked 15th among 25 industrial countries using different indicators.

Dr. Starfield and her colleagues took the study a step further. They considered and included adverse effects other than death in outpatient settings. Their findings are outlined below.

*Allan G. Hedberg, Ph.D.*

**MEDICAL ADVERSE EFFECTS IN OUTPATIENT SETTINGS:**

- 116 million extra physician visits
- 77 million extra prescriptions
- 17 million emergency department visits
- 8 million hospitalizations
- 3 million long-term admissions
- 199,000 additional deaths
- $77 billion in extra costs

Dr. Starfield profoundly observed that in her experience, most doctors are competent and genuinely concerned about the welfare of their patients. However, many are victimized by the deficiencies and the inefficiencies of our health care system just as are patients and their families. Physicians work with increased patient loads, mandated time line for patient visits, excessive paperwork, limitations on services rendered, delays in getting preauthorizations for treatment, denial of requested services. Further, errors occur as a result of increasing numbers of lawsuits or working under the threat of a lawsuit, and working with patients with whom there has not been an established bond of trust or a historical working relationship.

Dr. Starfield goes on to point out that the U.S. health industry is at risk due to the lack of a well-established primary care infrastructure.

What can the average patient and family member do in light of these findings to prevent any type of iatrogenic adverse side effect? Is it possible to identify several key steps that can be undertaken?

> **RECOMMENDED ACTIONS:**
>
> - When selecting a doctor or treatment program, scout around and compare until you are satisfied that you have selected a doctor in whom you have confidence and with whom you can communicate.
> - Ask questions until you are satisfied and understand the problem, the options for treatment, and that the best and most appropriate option has been selected.
> - Minimize hospitalizations and prolonged exposure to the hospital environment. Make frequent use of disinfectants commonly available in hospital settings such as canisters on the walls and available disinfectant bottles throughout the hospital.
> - Utilize alternatives to hospitalization and emergency room visits as much as possible.
> - Monitor progress and voice concern whenever there is doubt or a problem which appears to be emerging.
> - Be realistic, not obsessive-compulsive, irrational or delusional regarding germs, medical treatments, and health care environments.
> - Read on any procedure or treatment modality utilized so you know what can be expected and how to discuss with your health care provider any questions about the proposed procedure that you may have.

In brief, iatrogenic effects are unintended outcomes of treatment provided in a medical setting. While no one event or action may be the cause, they do happen. The prevention of such happenings is of prime importance to any and all medical professionals and the facilities within which services are rendered. Indeed, "an ounce of prevention is worth . . ." All of us need to do our part in reducing risk and helping bring about good treatment outcome and healthy lives.

# CHILDREN AND STRESS:
# HOW TO HELP YOUR CHILDREN COPE

Do children experience stress? Many people don't believe that they do; but perhaps those people don't know any children. Children know that they experience stress. What they often don't know is how to handle it.

Stress is an extra demand made on the body. Depending on the perceived danger or stress, our autonomic nervous system (that which governs involuntary actions) releases hormones causing chemical changes. Our hearts beat faster, our breathing speeds up, and blood flows into our brains. If we don't learn to deal with our stresses, we develop headaches, backaches, ulcers, heart attacks, and a whole list of annoying, damaging, and sometimes very serious problems.

Children are no different. If they are to survive and prosper in this world, they must know how to handle stress effectively.

How does your child handle stress? Think of a situation that your child has experienced as stressful, such as sharing his or her room with a sibling, canceling weekend plans, flunking a test, or not making the swim team.

Now think about how he or she reacted to that situation and choose one statement from below that best describes your child's reaction.

1. "Things like this always happen to me."
2. He or she acts unreasonably quiet and walks away.

3. "I never get what I want; you guys don't care about me," (is belligerent and verbally abusive).
4. "I am disappointed." (seconds later). "Oh well, maybe next time things will work out."
5. "This is no surprise; I was expecting it," (becoming withdrawn and preoccupied).
6. "That makes me angry but I didn't know what the difficulties were. What can I do to help?"
7. "That's not fair," (screaming and yelling).
8. Does not visibly react-withdraws and isolates himself or herself.

If you choose 4 or 6, your child is a capable kid. He or she handles stress well. A capable kid will express disappointment or anger and then quickly think of a way to feel better. Disappointment will last only a short time.

If you chose 1, 2, or 7, you have a slightly vulnerable child. Negative reactions were short-lived. The child soon calms down and becomes less preoccupied with himself or herself. While these children don't need professional help, they could benefit from learning more effective coping strategies such as how to relax, so that they aren't so reactive.

Selections 3, 5, or 8 indicate a seriously vulnerable child—possibly one who needs professional help. The response lasts longer than 24 hours, and he or she may display other negative behaviors.

Children who deal best with stress are those who have self-confidence and like themselves. The self-confident child stands straight, looks you in the eye, and talks competently and honestly about what he or she is doing. He or she is energetic, spontaneous, sensitive, and responsive to other people. When a crisis occurs, this child is reflective and helpful.

In my experience, children who handle stress the best have had parents or other adults in their lives who have given them the message: "You are a good person and I believe in you; even though

*Allan G. Hedberg, Ph.D.*

you make mistakes, my belief is that you will try to do better the next time." Children who receive this kind of message inevitably learn to believe in themselves. They know that whatever comes along, they can handle it because they have the internal resources to do so, or because they know where to go to get support and help. We can help our children deal with stress by letting them know that they have the capacity to handle whatever comes along.

How can parents convey this message to their children? There are many ways, but here are a few suggestions:

1. Treat your child with respect. Name-calling and angry words convey the message that the child is incapable, stupid or unlocked—and the child will believe this message.
2. When the child misbehaves, let him or her know that you disapprove of the behavior and follow through with reasonable consequences. Let the child know that you realize we all make mistakes and this is how we learn.
3. Express your love for your child through words and actions. Everyone needs to hear that he or she is loved, and we all need the physical warmth of a hug, a pat on the back, or the squeeze of a hand.

Enjoy being with your children! With mutual thought and discussion, you can find things to do together which are mutually enjoyable.

# Chapter Three

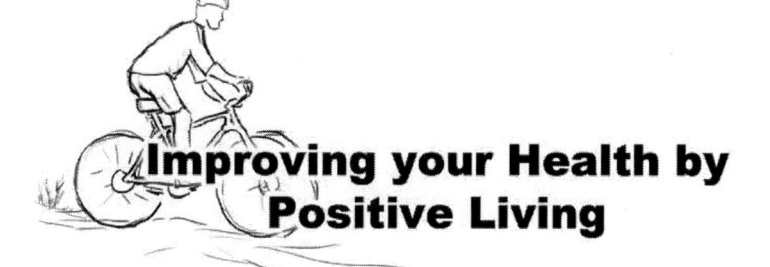

## Improving your Health by Positive Living

THE QUALITY OF LIFE IS DETERMINED BY ITS ACTIVITIES
*ARISTOTLE*

# THE IMPORTANCE OF GOOD COMMUNICATION

**INTRODUCTION**

Good communication facilitates the development of confidence, feelings of self-worth, and effective relationships with others. It makes life with those around us more pleasant and helps others develop good feelings about themselves and toward those with whom they associate in daily life.

Further, good communication facilities good health. Our communication style either creates stress for others and ourselves or it reduces the stress factor in our relationships. Stress is responsible for ill-health, ill-emotions and ill-thinking. Our physical, emotional, and mental health is directly affected by the way our speech imposes stress on ourselves and on another person.

Below are high stressful and low stressful styles of communication. Good communication skills generally contain low stressful styles of communication. It is important for all of us, but especially those in the public arena to study the chart below and practice the low stress communication style of speaking. At the same time one must avoid the high stressful styles of communication. The wellbeing and health of all parties will be affected accordingly. We all can change our style of communication and speak more freely and consistently in a low stress manner. To become more effective, select a few communication styles you would like to exhibit and practice speaking accordingly in that manner. Also select the communication patterns you need to stop expressing.

*Allan G. Hedberg, Ph.D.*

## HIGH STRESSFUL COMUNICATION STYLE

Monopolizing the conversation.

Interrupting.

Keeping a sour facial expression.

Withholding customary social cues such as greetings, nods, "uh-huh," and the like.

Throwing verbal barbs at others.

Using non-verbal put-downs.

Insulting or verbally abusing others.

Speaking dogmatically; not respecting others' opinions.

Complaining or whining excessively.

Criticizing excessively; fault finding.

Demanding one's own way; refusing to negotiate or compromise.

Ridiculing others.

Patronizing or talking down to others.

Making others feel guilty.

Losing one's temper frequently or easily.

Playing "games" with people; manipulating or competing in subtle ways.

Throwing "gotchas" at others.

Telling lies; evading honest questions.

Overusing "should" language.

Displaying frustration frequently.

Making aggressive demands of others.

Diverting conversation capriciously; breaking others' train of thought.

Disagreeing routinely.

Embarrassing or belittling others.

Asking loaded or accusing questions.

Overusing "why" questions.

Breaking confidences; failing to keep important promises.

Flattering others insincerely.

Joking at inappropriate times.

Bragging; talking only about self.

## LOW STRESSFUL COMMUNICATION STYLE

- Talking positively and constructively.
- Affirming feelings and needs of others.
- Stating one's needs and desires honestly.
- Leveling with others; sharing information and opinions openly and honestly.
- Confronting others constructively on difficult issues.
- Staying on the conversational topic until others have been heard.
- Stating agreement with others when possible.
- Questioning others openly and honestly; asking straight-forward, non-loaded questions.
- Keeping the confidences of others.
- Giving one's word sparingly and keeping it.
- Joking constructively and in good humor.
- Expressing genuine interest in the other person.
- Giving others a chance to express views or share information.
- Listening attentively; hearing other person out.
- Sharing one's thoughts and feelings with others.
- Giving positive non-verbal messages of acceptance and respect for others.
- Praising and complimenting others.
- Expressing respect for values and opinions of others.
- Giving suggestions constructively.
- Compromising; negotiating; helping others succeed.

Adapted from: Albrecht, K., *Stress and the Manager*, Prentice-Hall, 1979.

# THE ASSERTIVE OPTION OF COMMUNICATION

Have you ever had difficulty expressing your opinion in a group of friends or fellow workers? Was it difficult for you to be direct and clear in what you wanted to say?

Have you ever needed to give suggestions to or correct someone who was doing a poor job of typing, public relations, organizing an activity, or doing household repairs? Did you ignore the situation, hoping it would take care of itself? Did you come on too strong when you finally spoke up?

Do you self-consciously deny a sincerely expressed compliment? Do you respond to a compliment or statement of praise with humorous remarks that make the other person look foolish?

You probably have had to deal with at least one of these situations. Like most people, you probably felt trapped or restrained and unhappy with yourself in how you handled the situation, but thought that you had no other choice. When you felt this way, chances were you only had two options available. You could either respond passively or assertively.

You can say nothing at the time the situation occurred and simply ignore your feelings and even ignore the comment itself. This would be *passive or non-assertive behavior.* While it may prevent a conflict occurring with others, you probably will wind up feeling helpless, exploited, angry, ill, and disappointed with yourself. Also, you may lose the respect of others and, most importantly, lose respect for yourself.

The second option is *aggressive behavior*. You may use sarcasm and intimidations as your reaction without thinking. When you blow up at someone who isn't doing their work, you may not get the cooperation you want. When you belligerently complain about a neighbor's loud party, you may get them to quiet, but the relationship afterwards may have been jeopardized. You may actually feel uncomfortable or embarrassed with the way you acted.

There is a third option, one that is often overlooked. This is the *assertive behavior* option. The assertive option often helps people be true to themselves and achieve their goals without sacrificing important relationships. Acting assertively means standing up for your interpersonal rights and expressing what you believe or feel. When being assertive, you are direct, honest, and appropriate. You act in a manner that respects the rights of the other person. This is the most healthy communication pattern of the three.

Consider the tenets of assertive communication. Study them and learn how they apply to you. You could very well become more effective in your own sphere of relationships by being more consistently assertive.

> **TENNETS OF AN ASSERTIVE LIFESTYLE**
>
> 1. By standing up for ourselves and letting ourselves be known we gain self-respect and respect from other people.
> 2. By trying to live our lives in such a way that we never cause anyone to feel hurt under any circumstances, we end up hurting ourselves—and other people.
> 3. When we stand up for ourselves and express our honest feelings and thoughts in a direct and appropriate way, everyone usually benefits in the long run. Likewise, when we demean other people, we also demean ourselves and everyone involved usually loses in process.
> 4. By sacrificing our integrity and denying our personal feelings, relationships are usually damaged or prevented from developing. Likewise, personal relationships are damaged when we try to control others through hostility, intimidation or guilt.
> 5. Personal relationships become more authentic and satisfying when we share our true reactions with other people and do not block others' sharing their reactions with us.
> 6. Not letting others know what we think and feel is just as inconsiderate as not listening to other people's thoughts and feelings.
> 7. By acting assertively and telling people how their behavior affects us, we are giving them an opportunity to change their behavior, and we are showing respect for their right to know where they stand with us.

## Helping Yourself Accept Your Assertive Rights (Privileges)

Though other people may deny our right to speak up, many people find that the greater problem is within themselves. For instance, they may have been raised to believe that other people always come first. Consequently, they may have come to the conclusion that they are not good enough to have any rights as an individual. Having trouble accepting the fact that they do have assertive communication rights is not a sign of weakness. More often people do not speak out because they have learned to talk themselves out of public expression. Or, they may be surrounded by people who consistently deny that they have any rights to assertively speak and represent a given point of view. They may even forego any and every opportunity to speak up.

You can help yourself by accepting your right to be understood by following these four steps:

- Step One: Become aware of the internal messages you give yourself that cause you to believe that you aren't entitled to rights.
- Step Two: Develop more realistic messages that you can use to counter your rights-denying message.
- Step Three: Repeatedly practice internally giving yourself the counter-message. Having others say that you have rights or reading books that confirm your rights is a helpful middle step. Ultimately, you need to be able to give yourself these messages.
- Step Four: In small appropriate ways, act on your right to speak up while internally affirming to your right to do so.

Remember, you have a choice to exercise your assertive option or not, as situations change. Remembering that you have this choice allows you the freedom to increase your interpersonal effectiveness and your general health and wellbeing.

# SMOKE NO MORE: PREPARING FOR A SMOKELESS LIFE

Smoking is the #1 preventable cause of disease and breakdown within the heart, lungs, lips, palate, stomach, kidneys, and bladder. A cigarette is not a health food. Yet, despite dire warnings, over 100,000,000 Americans continue to puff away. Most smokers live a life of conflict and dilemma. While they often find smoking to be pleasing to the sense and enjoyable, they also live with a constant desire and preference to stop smoking. Those who quit, do so because of personal and family concerns, vanity and progressive symptoms of ill health. For you, this may be your day of decision. Make a life decision. Go for it!

Research findings indicate that 68% of smokers say they would like to quit smoking. Of those that did try to quit, about 65% did so without medication or cessation counseling. Over the past 10 years, more smokers than ever engage in some type of program or plan to quit. You can be one of them. Go for it!

Giving up cigarette smoking cannot be undertaken lightly, and should be done deliberately. Impulsive, dramatic "crash" programs to quit are rarely successful. Success requires careful thought and planning, and adequately preparing yourself both physically and psychologically. It would be important to remember that some sacrifices and concessions to your normal daily routine must be made, however, they are only temporary. Set your mind and focus on the rewards awaiting you in this venture. The following suggestions will lessen the periods of sacrifice, inconvenience, and will maximize success:

1. **Decide which method of quitting is best for you.** "Cold turkey" has been successfully used by many. It is a sudden, complete break from cigarettes. "Tapering off" is having the goal of gradually reducing your cigarette consumption either to zero, or to half your daily quota, and then stopping completely.
2. **Determine a specific quitting day, "Q-Day."** Consider a date that will include a time period as free of personal tension producing problems as possible; a time when your social calendar can spare you from gatherings where smoking prevails. Keep yourself in smoke-free environments,
3. **If you opt for "tapering off," the following may be helpful:** a) Each time your reach for a cigarette, ask yourself if you really need it. You may learn that many cigarettes are merely a reflex action, lit without regard for conscious need. b) Decide arbitrarily that you will smoke only on the odd or even numbered hours of the clock. c) Be selective in your choice of certain cigarettes that seem more important to you than others. Also, it may help to switch brands during this period.
4. **To better help you, give proper attention to emergencies and be prepared with counter measures.** a) Put all cigarettes, ash trays, matches and lighters out of arm's way. b) Have on hand a plentiful supply of fresh fruits and snacks, which could include olives, celery, carrots, crackers, mints, gum, etc. c) Reading, crossword puzzles, and other similar activities that keep your hands busy are also helpful. Relax!
5. **Plan to go to bed earlier and get up earlier for a few days.** This will help you avoid the tension of hurrying through breakfast and rushing to work. Take naps during the day whenever possible as the impulse to smoke during sleep is a rare occurrence. Use deep breathing techniques. Slow inhalation and exhalation.

Never wait until panic strikes before you start to think about what to do. You must be ready in advance to meet emergencies. The above

*Allan G. Hedberg, Ph.D.*

preparations and suggestions are designed to help you start your stop smoking program with a head start. Share your plan to stop smoking with someone who will hold you accountable and who will be a source of encouragement.

# SLEEP IMPROVES HEALTH AND PERFORMANCE

Sleep is one of the primary contributors to wellness. One can get along reasonably well without a positive sleep pattern for several days, but after that the absence of sleep or restless sleep begins to take its toll. Sleep, or the lack of it, has a profound effect upon our cognitive processing of information and our general levels of restlessness, irritability, and alertness. Sleep patterns also affect our interpersonal relationships.

In a recent research study of Law Enforcement Officers, it was found that 40% reported a pattern of sleep disturbance. The study also found a correlation between sleep problems and making administrative errors, fatigue, sleeping while driving or in meetings, citizen's complaints, absenteeism, anger, depression and other moods. The research was conducted by Dr. Shantha Rajaratnam of the Brigham and Women's Hospital, Boston.

If a poor sleep pattern develops, it needs to be addressed in an assertive and forth right matter, preferably without the use of sleeping medication. If sleep medication is required, it is best to use it for a short period of time, such as several weeks to several months. Use it periodically as needed rather than routinely.

Addressing sleep behaviorally is the best approach for long-term benefit. Below are sleep related conditions that might be tried and utilized. It is best to try one of the suggestions for at least one to two weeks before deciding if it is going to be helpful or not.

First, the general self-control pattern for insomnia is as follows: If you're awakened at night, deeply relax in bed for a while in the hopes that sleep will return. If not, don't just lie there and grow tense and frustrated, but get out of bed and do some quiet activity such as reading or listening to the radio or finishing a project until you feel sleepy once again. At that point return to bed. If you are not sleeping within 15-20 minutes, get out of bed and repeat this process as often as necessary every night for at least 30 nights.

Sleep patterns can be changed and improved. It takes however, a very concerted and intentional approach over an extended period of time.

The following sleep enhancing suggestions have been put forth by a sleep researcher, Dr. Peter Hauri, in an article published in Psychology Today in June, 1986. Try each of the below suggestions for at least 7-10 nights before discarding any of them.

**Dr. Hauri's Sleep Strategies**

- If you are awakened during the night, relax in bed for a while and let sleep return. Try reading or listening to music. If this doesn't work and you grow tense and frustrated, get out of bed and do some quiet activity until you're sleepy once again, then return to bed. Repeat this as often as necessary.
- The most crucial rule: Never oversleep because of a poor night's sleep. If you are under age 50 get up at the same time every morning. This sets the body's internal sleep/wake clock.
- Try to set a regular bedtime, but delay it if necessary so you go to bed only when tired and sleep can overtake you.
- Cut down on alcohol, smoking, chocolate, coffee, tea and caffeinated soft drinks; avoid them in the afternoon or evening or eliminate them if you're sensitive to them.
- Schedule time in the early evening to write down worries or concerns and what you will do about them the next day.
- Experiment with your bedroom's noise level and temperature and find what's best for you.

*Achieving and Living a Healthy Lifestyle in a World of Stress*

- Avoid heavy meals too close to bedtime and eating in the middle of the night. But a midnight snack of hot milk and crackers has been said to help some people sleep.
- Stay fit with regular exercise, but not too close to bedtime.
- Keep physically active if possible the day after a bad night's sleep and avoid napping unless you are certain that naps will help you sleep on the following night.
- Learn relaxation techniques such as progressively tightening and releasing muscles, visualizing peaceful scenes or doing boring mental tasks.
- Find out if medical conditions or prescription drugs, including pain pills, could be keeping you awake.
- Get professional help in coping with life stresses or learn biofeedback or other types of stress management techniques.

Goodnight and have a good sleep. See you in the morning . . .

# REAL MEN COPE WELL

Throughout the history of research, we have consistently studied the differences between men and women in personality patterns, how they process information, react to situations, and live their daily lives. Our research has revealed certain patterns in which men have certain advantages in some areas while women have certain advantages in other areas. Often, no strong differences are found. A book was published a few years ago summarizing the differences between men and women on a host of research studies. The implication of the differences was discussed.

Political correctness tries to provide equal provisions, programs and services for men and women. This viewpoint, however, defies the research findings on the inherent distinctions of the very nature between men and women. For example, this viewpoint is responsible for the closing of private boy's schools despite their very high success rate when girls are not allowed to enroll.

Similarly, the Christian church and other religious faiths have targeted men for specialized ministries over the past decade or two and are developing authentic masculine participation options. Promise Keepers is one such example. The book by John Eldredge (Thomas Nelson, 2001) entitled, *Wild At Heart*, speaks of a masculinity movement within the church aimed to attract men to church by changing the church atmosphere. Further, the Biblical image of Jesus as a strong man and leader is being rekindled.

## THE MALE IDENTITY-A WORK IN PROGRESS

The brains of men and women function differently. In fact, recent research has noted that there is a huge difference between the processing of information in a man's and in a woman's brain. Typically, a woman's brain is very active. It is always working. Thinking, planning, preparing, especially in the emotional part of the brain. The man's brain, by comparison, is relatively quiet. It needs stimulation. We see this difference particularly in the aging brains of men and women.

An article in *Livescience* by Geanna Bryner, states that, "men are more likely than women to have problems with memory and other thinking skills." As aging increases into the years of 70 and beyond, men are one and a half times more likely to have mild cognitive impairment than women. The male brain ages much more rapidly than women's brain. While the male brain seems to age more rapidly, the disorder of Alzheimer's seems to set in at a higher percentage level for women, however. Research is ongoing in this area of study.

These findings tend to suggest that men cope with stress, trauma, and difficult situations in their life differently from women due to a different neurological structure and process. Simply stated, men tend to forget the negative events in their life where women tend to rehearse, refocus, and retain the emotional memory of negative events in their life. As a result, women may tend to suffer more from negative events due to this enhanced and prolonged memory of negative events.

In contrast, social learning theorists contend that we learn attitudes and behavioral patterns as a consequence of the ways in which we are rewarded and punished. We learn how to behave, how to think, what to expect from others, and how to deal with stress and trauma as a result of what we see and hear in the world around us. We tend to imitate what is effectively modeled before us. Rewards, punishments and behavioral models come into our daily lives in a multitude of subtle, blatant, and ingenuous forms. For example, our social identity is strongly influenced from the television programs we watch, magazine ads, physical punishment during childhood, fairy tale stories, public images, memberships in clubs and organizations, how we are touched by others, epitaphs, as well as terms of endearment expressed to us over our life span. Experiencing such events differently, boys learn to behave in a unique way compared to girls in how they use their cognitive skills, develop expectations from life, and how they cope with success and failure.

Further, cognitive theorists argue that sex roles are acquired at specific developmental learning stages during childhood. Throughout life, we change in our viewpoint of what is appropriate and inappropriate as a boy or as a girl. Gender identity commences around age 3 and continues to do so for the next few years as boys identify themselves in comparison to girls. What follows is a developmental gender driven desire for the specific rewards associated with being a boy or a girl. Maleness, for a boy, becomes instilled as the choice or option to do "boy things" is rewarded. Rewarding girls for doing "girl things," therefore results in the development of a young lady with associated behavioral patterns. Even the way in which we handle stress and trauma follows gender identity. Being rewarded for gender relevant and appropriate patterns of behavior in dealing with stress is basic to our self-identity and social skill development. As we develop, we increasingly select patterns of behavior which are identified with the prevailing male or female image in our culture. As we are rewarded in accordance with our gender, we refine our sexuality and gender identity.

## FOUR CASE STUDIES

While there are a number of stressors that men face, they do cope with them in their own way, often in ways that are unhealthy. For example, men have particular difficulty facing and confronting loss in their life. For example:

1. Bill lost his wife through death related to Congestive Heart Failure. He was devastated and depressed. He struggled.

Alcohol and long hours of sleeping became his avoidance pattern. He was not able to find a healthy pattern of living for over five years following the death of his wife. Finally, he recovered and moved forward in his life after seeking personal counseling.

2. Frank lost the intimate companionship and sexual gratification when his wife underwent a double mastectomy. While still being sexually motivated and active he went off the deep end and sought comfort from prostitutes and single women he met in the bars he frequented. He not only lost perspective but, eventually, lost his wife totally to divorce when she could take his philandering no more.

3. Carlos was not able to handle the loss of his baby when at 18 years of age, his girlfriend became pregnant and, subsequently, decided to abort the child without consulting him and without his consent. The loss was a personal and deep blow. He was devastated by the loss of his child and not being consulted about his wishes for the child's birth and future welfare. Carlos became angry, aggressive and combative with his girlfriend. His relationship with his employer and friends became impaired. His own family went through enormous amount of suffering until they finally confronted him about such behavior. Through personal therapy he and his family learned of his deep remorse and anger over the loss of his child that he dearly wanted to rear and make part of his life.

4. Leo worked for a local manufacturing company. He was assigned a particular piece of equipment to operate. He soon realized that it was unsafe. He told his supervisor three times about the danger and how the equipment could be modified to make it safe. His pleadings were ignored. A month after his third pleading, his arm became caught in the equipment. It was literally torn from the socket of the elbow. For the three years following the loss of his arm, even though he had a prosthetic device, he did not go out in public. In social situations he would cover the arm with a long-sleeved shirt or coat, or attempt to hide it under the other arm by folding his arms in front of him. He was socially

embarrassed despite the fact that he knew he was not the one responsible for the loss of his arm. He became angry and bitter. He did not learn to live with the prosthetic arm and remained embarrassed by it. He coped by withdrawing, isolating, avoiding, and displaced aggression. Finally, after four years he sought counseling and significantly benefited. Life took a positive turn.

---

**THE NINE MOST STRESSFUL LIFE CHANGING EVENTS**
1. Death of a spouse.
2. Marital separation/divorce.
3. Death of a close friend or family member.
4. Personal injury or illness.
5. Marriage.
6. Fired at work.
7. Retirement.
8. Business readjustment.
9. Change in financial status.

---

## COPING STRATEGIES

As we can see, exposure to such extraordinary stressful and catastrophic events induces a biopsychological process that is reactive and transformative in nature. How a man reacts and copes with such situations determines the extent of the impact of the trauma in all areas of his life. Coping style also depends upon gender, as well as age, race, and previous experience with stress and trauma. Men tend to focus on those coping strategies that quickly reduce their anxiety, fear, guilt, shame and emotional hurt. Men desire a quick resolution.

We refer to the self protective strategies as defense mechanisms, some of which are unhealthy and some healthy. Further, several of the most common unhealthy and healthy ways of coping are listed below:

## Unhealthy Ways Of Coping

Just what are the reasons men tend to cope with harmful events in life in unhealthy ways? Here are a few examples of why men utilize dysfunctional coping styles.

1. Men are less socially connected than women. When stress and difficulties come into the life of a man, most likely he does not have a strong social network on which to rely and obtain support. Essentially, men go it alone.
2. When pressure builds and difficulties in life emerge, men tend to avoid the situation rather than to deal with it in an open and direct manner. For instance, men drink much more alcohol under stress than women. Not only is the alcohol consumption unhealthy, but the avoidance of the stressful circumstance allows the problem to linger and develops into an unhealthy habit of behavior.
3. Men tend to take risks and place themselves in even greater stressful and dangerous situations. As a result, they place their bodies and emotions at increased risk rather than lowering their risk status by problem solving. This increases an unhealthy lifestyle status. Their body takes a toll. This type of coping style can be self-defeating and self-destructive.
4. Men prefer not to seek professional counsel but take the approach of an individualist when stressed or traumatized. They do not seek the counsel of therapists or physicians as do women. Men do not connect as do women with a social network or a religious and faith-building network of a local church. Nor do men utilize religious or self-help reading material for guidance when distressed.

*Allan G. Hedberg, Ph.D.*

## Healthy Ways Of Coping

The ability to regulate stress, anger, pain and trauma has an important and positive bearing on a man's human relations performance and job satisfaction. It is vital for men to learn positive strategies and not over-react to stressful traumatic events and impair his marriage, family life, job and his community involvements. Repeated stressful provocation without resolution also increases susceptibility to hypertension, physical and mental ailments, and other disabling physical and medical conditions. Just what are some healthy and positive strategies of coping with trauma?

1. Learn to relax when stressed through deep breathing, visual imagery, aerobic exercises, anerobic exercises and reading.
2. Do not drink alcohol or reduce the amount consumed when stressed.
3. Sleep at least eight hours nightly at times of stress. A 1-hour power nap during the day can be helpful.
4. Take vitamins and eat a balanced meal especially vegetables and fruits when under stress.
5. Talk, talk, talk. Tell the story of the stressful event, your feelings about it, how it seems to be affecting you, what you want to do about it, and what you want to come out of it.
6. Manage your time for work, personal demands, relaxation and recreational activities.
7. Believe that a positive and optimistic viewpoint can moderate stress. Gain a realistic and positive perspective of any stressful situation.
8. Spend more time with uplifting, reassuring, comforting, and problem solving friends.
9. Seek the advice of a professional therapist. In so doing, the problem may be addressed and new skills may be learned.
10. Reclaim your childhood faith to gain an optimistic perspective, personal meaning, self-worth, and a sense of benevolence whenever trauma strikes.

## UNHEALTHY DEFENSE STRATEGIES

1. Repression—Pushing away from awareness any painful event and thought.
2. Denial—Refusing to accept certain facts or statements as true.
3. Regression—Return to an earlier stage of development in reaction to a threatening act or situation.
4. Reaction Formation—Replacing of a negative feeling such as anxiety with the opposite feeling or developing an impairment that prevents engaging in an anxiety activity.
5. Projection—Attributing one's own feelings to other people rather than claiming responsibility oneself.
6. Displacement—Attributing a negative experience to some other source as in blaming others for the circumstance.
7. Rationalization—Creating a false believable rationale, opinion or course of action to justify a wrongful behavior, opinion, or decision.

*Allan G. Hedberg, Ph.D.*

---

**HEALTHY DEFENSE STRATEGIES**

1. Reconciliation—Coming together of two or more people with differences and re-establishing broken relationships on new terms.
2. Forgiveness—Accepting responsibility for one's own actions and seeking reconciliation with another by ceasing the unwanted behavior that caused the hurt.
3. Assertiveness—Openly and forthrightly speaking to the truth of a matter while being considerate and without being verbally aggressive towards the other person.
4. Accommodation—Making reasonable adjustments to a situation that cannot be changed as in learning to live with it or beyond it
5. Compromise—Reaching some mutually agreeable stance with another person in which both individuals accept an agreement on terms that are less than preferred by both parties.
6. Consideration—Listening empathically to the story of another person who feels hurt, offended, or unjustly treated, followed by compassionate support and care.

---

## STRESS INOCULATION

Policemen, firemen and military personnel are high stress occupations that benefit from stress inoculation training. Such professionals absorb frustration and hostility more than others. However, all men have a degree of provocation proneness and could benefit from stress inoculation training as well.

As the name suggests, the procedure of inoculation training entails the acquisition of healthy skills that enable a person to cope effectively with stressful, painful, hurtful, or traumatic situations. Analogs to medical inoculation, a man's resistance to stress is enhanced by a regulated pre-exposure to stress events such that his emotional reactions aroused but not overwhelmed when stress is encountered any time thereafter. Inoculation training has three stages:

1. **An educational phase** which provides an educational framework for a man to understand stress and his typical emotional and physical response to stressful events. For example, a CPA is taught to monitor the buildup of stress symptoms as April, 15$^{th}$ approaches, namely, hypertension, irritability, tension, insomnia, short temper, headaches, body sweating, backaches, conflict and clenching of the jaw.
2. **A rehearsal phase** which provides specific healthy cognitive and behavioral coping techniques for a man to learn and utilize. For example, as stress signs develop, he is taught to breathe deep, relax the muscles, use calming imagery, express relaxing phrases, engage in positive self-talk, and talk assertively.
3. **An application phase** which gives the man an opportunity to become proficient in the effective coping skills noted above by practicing them under regulated mild stressful conditions. For example, the CPA is taught the above stress management skills during December through February so he can make full use of these newly learned stress reduction skills during March and April when on the job stress is at its greatest level and he is at risk for illness and relationship problems with clients, family and colleagues.

## PUTTING IT ALL TOGETHER

Real men cope well. Real men think ahead and learn healthy and effective coping strategies. They learn to communicate. They learn when to let go of something and to no longer harbor a grudge or ill content. They learn how and when to relax and let go of stress and tension. They do not abuse alcohol. They develop positive and optimistic ways of thinking and dealing with circumstances in their life. They realize that defeat does not come from events that happen, but from how they respond or choose not to respond to situations

*Allan G. Hedberg, Ph.D.*

that happen. Real men cope well through spending time with uplifting, positive, and supportive friends and associates. They are open to seeking advice from others, especially from professionals. And, they develop within themselves a deep, personal and living faith.

Real men cope well. They prepare ahead. Real men undergo the process of inoculation to stress events in life. They prepare ahead. They educate themselves, they read, they study, they discuss, they consider, and they share with others. They learn and rehearse skills that will help them cope with unplanned trauma. They are ready to take whatever comes, deal with it forthrightly, and learn from it secondarily. As a result they become better men, husbands, fathers and business partners.

Real men cope well. They teach others what they have learned from loss, failure, disappointment, hurt, and defeat, to name a few of life's learning experiences. They pass along their stories of what happened to them and what they did to overcome successfully. They teach their children, spouse, associates, friends and their community by their lifestyle example.

# LOVING HOMES, HEALTHIER CHILDREN

Children who believe their parents love them tend to be healthier as adults. It may not matter as much as to how parents convey their love or if the love is manifest in a very strong and consistent manner, so long as the children in the home believe or perceive their parents do love them.

In 1950, psychological researchers from the University of Arizona interviewed eighty-seven undergraduates at Harvard University and then followed up with a second interview thirty-five years later. The students who gave their parents high ratings for loving characteristics showed levels of disease far lower than the students who rated their parents low on the love scale. Dr. Gary Schwartz of the University of Arizona was the lead researcher of the study.

In the research, other factors were ruled out that might explain the correlation, including family history of disease, the death or divorce of parents, marital and smoking history of the subjects, and socio-economic factors.

Dr. Schwartz and his associate, Dr. Linda Russek, stated that the perception of love and caring may serve as a buffer against the stresses of everyday life which often affect one's long-term health.

The students in the study scored their parents on a scale from 1 to 9 on the characteristics of loving, just, fair, clever, hard-working, and strong. These characteristics fell into two primary categories, love and wisdom, and basic caring. Of the 87 students interviewed, 19 of the students rated their parents low in both of these categories. Thirty-five years later, 84% of the 19 students were diagnosed with diseases such as cardiovascular disorders, ulcers, and alcoholism. Forty-one of the students rated their parents high on both categories. Only 37% of the 41 students were diagnosed with diseases thirty-five years later.

To be sure, one of the primary messages to remember about this research is that parental love really matters in the life of children, says Dr. Schwartz.

# INTERPERSONAL RELATIONSHIPS AFFECT HEALTH

Healthy interpersonal relationships are essential to healthy lives. We gain strength and support from our relationships, and we meet our basic needs for belonging and value through our relationships. Friends do make good medicine, both preventative and corrective.

On the other hand, interpersonal relationships inevitably become entangled in unresolvable conflict. For some of us, that conflict comes from within our immediate family, from extended family members, or from those with whom we work. Unfortunately, we usually become involved in conflict out of the experiences we have with our most significant relationships. Marital dissolution, child custody and visitation problems, or even work-related events, such as wrongful termination, harassment, and other traumatic events are a few examples. Conflict saps energy, diverts attention, and reduces performance. Conflict creates a wedge between ourselves and the very people who are our primary source of personal support.

We each have our own style of responding to conflict. Some of us avoid. Others of us attack. Still others deny. And others try to compromise. Below is a short quiz to give you an estimate of your conflict resolution style. Select the answer most likely to represent your response in the situations presented. Your answer will indicate your tendency to <u>avoid</u>, <u>attack</u>, <u>deny</u>, <u>accommodation</u>, or <u>compromise</u> when facing conflict.

1. a) I try to avoid creating unpleasantness for myself. (Avoid/Deny)
   b) I try to win my position. (Attack)

2. a) I am usually firm in pursuing my goals. (Attack)
   b) I attempt to get all concerns and issues immediately out in the open. (Accommodation)

3. a) I propose a middle ground. (Compromise)
   b) I press to get my points made. (Attack)

4. a) I try to find a compromise solution. (Compromise)
   b) I attempt to deal with all of their and my concerns. (Accommodation)

5. a) I try to seek a way to get along with the opposing party by accommodations to their views over my own. (Accommodation)
   b) I try to find some aspect of the opposing party's views that I can live with through compromise. (Compromise)

## Tips for Controlling Anger

Before the next argument or conflict develops in which you are a primary participant or an observer, approach it with a pre-learned anger control strategy. For example, consider and adopt for your regular use one of the following two acronyms:

### RID

R   Recognize the anger signals or cues that preceded the conflict and that are present at the time the conflict became expressed.
I   Identify positive ways to think about the situation that has developed.
D   Do something constructive to calm down and approach the situation rationally.

## RESOLVED

**R** Relax yourself before you enter into any dialogue with others in the dispute.
**E** Expect that you will be treated with respect and that an answer can be reached.
**S** State the problem as objectively and behaviorally as you can, from your point of view.
**O** Open the discussion to obtain the viewpoints of all the persons involved.
**L** List the possible solutions together.
**V** Veto the solutions that are unacceptable or undesirable to anyone involved in the conflict.
**E** Evaluate the relative merits of the remaining solutions.
**D** Develop the most acceptable solution to all parties concerned.

There are a number of other strategic steps that can be taken to achieve a peaceful resolution of a conflict. However, a systematic approach must be followed for any problem to be effectively resolved.

In summary, relationships usually rise or fall on the presence or absence of conflict and how we proceed to resolve any conflict that exists. Our personal effectiveness in our relationships is directly related to how conflict is handeled. If we do not have a natural manner in dealing with conflict, we need to learn how to do so. The sooner the better as conflict is inevitable.

# IN SEARCH OF THE HEALTHY FAMILY

Delores Curran, a syndicated columnist, authored a significant book entitled, <u>Traits of a Healthy Family,</u> Winston Press. Serving as the foundation of this book were the responses of 500 social workers, educators, family therapists, and church workers to a questionnaire sent to solicit their views on the healthy family. These respondents were asked to select fifteen traits commonly found among families that they know and consider to be healthy.

In viewing the answers of these 500 professionals, it was found that, first and foremost, today's healthy family communicates and listens. Clearly, communication is the key to a strong family. "Healthy families listen responsively rather than reactively. They pay attention to non-verbal communication, particularly silences and touches, "says Curran.

The author's research also revealed that "Healthy families quarrel, but rapidly find their way to reconciliation through communication. On the other hand, the non-healthy families tend to let quarrels continue without making up. This produces hurts and withdrawal from each other.

## Healthy Traits

What are the other traits associated with strong and healthy families? Below is the list of the 15 positive traits generated by these 500 professionals. Evaluate the family in which you were raised. Evaluate the family life you are now creating as a parent and/or family member.

- Affirmation and mutual support.
- A balance self-esteem.
- Respect for individual differences.
- A high sense of trust.
- A sense of shared responsibility.
- Teach right from wrong.
- Family life with many traditions.
- A sense of play and humor.
- A balance of interaction among members.
- A shared religious/spiritual faith.
- A respect for one another's privacy.
- Place value on service to others.
- Foster table time conversation.
- Share leisure time together.
- Admit to and seek help with problems.

## The Challenge

The above traits represent a challenge to <u>every</u> family. While no one family would conceivably possess all these healthy traits, they do represent guidelines or objectives for each family to develop. They encompass the relationships that prevail across generations. The degree to which these traits are learned gives any family a rich heritage of memories. The traits outlined also give strength to face the stresses of day-to-day living by each family member. The process is dynamic and ongoing. Go for it!

# HEALTHY LIVING TAKES TIME

The Canadian Broadcasting Corporation and the Canadian Heart and Stroke Foundation conducted an online survey recently and concluded that 2,160 Canadians adults did not have time for healthy living. They did not have time to exercise or to eat healthy meals. Granted, healthy meals may take longer to prepare and eat. At the same time, the responding Canadians acknowledged that heart disease and stroke can be fought by making healthy behavioral choices. Obviously, knowledge is one thing while behavior is another. Apparently, the twain does not meet.

Further, there was another distressing disconnect in the answers of the respondents. While they responded correctly to a series of questions about heart disease and strokes, they were not doing the appropriate actions to prevent and protect themselves from heart disease and stroke.

In reviewing the results of the survey, many excuses were given as to the reason for being unhealthy even though they knew better. Time was the primary excuse. For example, 44% of the respondents said they had no time for regular physical activity. 41% said healthy meals were too complex and took too long to prepare. 51% said that fast food outlets do not have enough healthy choices. 31% said that the time they would like to spend being active was actually spent commuting. These findings are important to consider since heart disease and stroke causes about one in three Canadians to die, and are the leading killers of women.

The antidote proposed in this research was that of less television watching among other action steps. It was found that 25% of Canadians over 20 years of age spent two hours a day or more watching television. Other ways to devote time for healthy living include, working less over-time, generating a contract with yourself to devote an hour a day to engage in health improvement activities, and establishing a buddy-system with a friend to undertake more healthy activities daily.

Healthy living is a matter of priority and choice. It is possible to live healthier and enjoy the benefits of healthy living, but it takes time, intentionality, and persistence. These traits are learned and acquired and followed. May we take the challenge?

# HAPPINESS AND OPTIMISM: THE POSITIVE ALTERNATIVE LIFESTYLE

Throughout the annals of human history, fields of psychology, psychiatry, and other associated professions have focused on mental illness and the repair of psychological and emotional damage. Diagnostic procedures, treatment methods, rehabilitation, specialized language, and theory development have all focused on what has gone wrong. Understanding human weakness, preventing sickness, and rebuilding the lost human spirit have been the historical hallmarks of psychology and psychiatry.

In the mid-1990's, through the creative work of Dr. Martin Seligman and others, we began to look at the other side of the coin—the side of strength, the side of what people do well and are good at. Positive psychology has now been coined and has become the new direction. Positive psychology is the scientific pursuit of optimal human functioning and the building of human strength and virtue. It is the focus of understanding, prevention of illness and promotion of health.

Positive psychology is currently percolating into the way medical practitioners approach treatment. We are now seeing its application in business, education, sports programs, and health-care research, to name a few areas of development.

Through the framework of positive psychology, we have discovered that there is a set of human strengths that buffer against mental illness. These strengths include courage, optimism, personal skill, work ethic, hope, honesty, and perseverance. Positive psychology has become a science of human strength whose mission is to foster positive virtues in young people who will live them out during their adult years. The objective is that our youth will become a positive benefactor of such human virtues, which will then benefit those in the community and others whose lives they will ultimately touch. Positive psychology is a shift in focus—from decreasing one's deviance from a healthy condition to increasing one's existing potential strengths. It is the discovery and development of our hidden talents within each of us that enable us to thrive.

It is important to understand and accept the basic premise of positive psychology: We come to be who we are through the social learning process. We learn to walk, to run, and skip. We learn to speak our native language by imitating those around us. We learn to treat people respectfully by being respected and imitating respectful behavior. We learn to solve problems. We learn to resolve conflict. Life is itself the summation and the integration of learned behavioral patterns to which we have ascribed meaning, purpose, and future direction.

Happiness and optimism are two key learned behavioral patterns. They are developed experientially and progressively. It is essential to train ourselves to be happy and optimistic individuals. Only then will we be able to experience a contented life, a deeper sense of peace and have a buffer against mental illness.

## The Three Components of Happiness

The root of positive psychology contains the basic ways that we ordinarily look at life and acquire the behaviors we desire to experience each day. Unfortunately, many of us may not have been trained to create happiness or well-being or even recognize it when it is happening. There are three components to a life of happiness and satisfaction. The three components are characterized by the common verbal exchanges we have with other people, i.e., "Have a good day," "Hope you're having a pleasant day," and "Did you have a meaningful experience today?"

*Allan G. Hedberg, Ph.D.*

When we exchange greetings with others and wish them a good day, essentially we are focusing on having a good day ourselves and wanting others to experience a good day also. For most of us, a *good* day is associated with the absence of a stressful event. When we have a *pleasant* day, we generally refer to a day of fun, enjoyment, and relaxation. When we speak of a *meaningful* day, we refer to activities of helping others, reflection, or a spiritual encounter.

## Hazel's Story

Hazel Woodgreen resides in a skilled nursing facility. She is from the east coast but came to California for her last years to be near her daughter. Hazel is in the beginning stages of dementia; however, she still has good long-term memory.

In speaking with her regarding her personal history, she made three profound statements. All three are indicative of a positive personality and attitude.

Hazel stated, "I lived a good life. It was marked with love, engagement, compassion, and it was very satisfying." Second, she stated, "My husband was a very pleasant man and we had a pleasant marriage together." She went on to say, "We had fun together. We would often go for dinner and dancing, and enjoyed our family life together. We had a life of healthy living, and we savored positive feelings." Third, she said, "I always tried to be of help to others." She continued by recounting the many organizations that she helped in her community as a volunteer. This was her way to give back something larger and more permanent than herself. Interestingly, she had two other female roommates who were experiencing dementia and benefited from Hazel's willingness to help them be more comfortable as the need arose.

## Weekly Happiness Exercises

There are many ways people go about the learning process to increase their level of happiness. The following exercises suggest a few ways people have learned to experience happiness. Try them out for yourself. Select one exercise each day and soon it will become a routine lifestyle. The sooner you begin, the better. Teach them to your children by example and intentional practice. For example:

1. Express your gratitude to someone who has touched and enriched your life in the past.
2. Give yourself a beautiful day by appreciating and indulging in that which gives you pleasure.
3. Increase positive meaning in your life by engaging in something you believe in and is larger than yourself.
4. Respond actively to a positive event that has come to your attention.
5. Be friendly to someone each day; you will in turn gain a friend.
6. Become associated with a challenging situation and work to make that situation better and successful.
7. Become aware that God is doing something amazing. Exercise your faith and find out what you can do to become part of the action.
8. Write a gratitude journal each week by writing down three to five things for which you are thankful.
9. Practice a random or specific act of kindness by doing a kind thing for family, friends, and/or strangers.
10. Let go of anger and resentment by writing a letter of forgiveness to a person who has hurt or wronged you in the past.
11. Write a statement about a time you were at your best; then reflect on the personal strength you displayed at that time.
12. Identify what you consider to be your top five strengths. Then make use of one of the top five strengths in a new and different way each day for the next week.

13. Teach children to live, cope, and relate to others with a "happy heart."

## The Principle of Optimism

In addition to happiness, positive psychology, according to Dr. Robert Kokoska, underscores the principle of optimism. It is considered a cherished positive parameter of human excellence. It is generally considered that optimistic people are usually happier and more highly productive than pessimists. Optimism, like happiness, can be taught and learned. According to the new thinking of positive psychology, there tends to be a healthy and upward flow of achievements in those people who are highly optimistic and cheerful. This positive flow of success usually causes a person to be tougher mentally and psychologically.

For some of us, unfortunately, trauma and tragedy have come into our lives. The noxious efforts of tragedy often lead to a sense of self-defeating attitudes and behavior. The end is self-destruction. However, according to Dr. Paul Wong of Tyndale College, "If we have learned the value of hope against all odds, we can affirm the positive in all extremely negative circumstances." This is known as Tragic Optimism. Armed with the viewpoint we can be optimistic even when facing tragedy. With optimism, we can believe and know with assurance that help is on the way, that there is always the hope of restoration, and that we can become a better person out of a painful ordeal.

## Weekly Optimism Exercises

1. Look for something of value in each and every circumstance of life.
2. Express optimistic statements daily to your children and others.

3. When something goes wrong or sour, examine it to see if the situation could have been avoided or changed had you been optimistic from the start.
4. Develop optimistic strategies for coping with stress and hardship. Quote axioms to yourself, such as, "This too shall pass" or "That which doesn't kill me makes me stronger."
5. When others around you undergo tragedy, consider what one could be optimistic about in the situation and for the future.
6. Write down five things you hope for and want to occur over the coming month.
7. When you want something you can not have, think on five things you do have.

## Summary

In summary, human psychology always has been a study of negative human behavior and, as a result, has been often regarded negatively by a segment of society. Basically, psychology has been perceived as a sign of trouble, and, thus, attempts have been made to correlate it to such destructive human experiences like depression, psychosis, unhappiness, mental disorders, and trauma. Sadly, most of the clinical examinations also have tended to look at a disorder as a sickness or a weakness. Most of the treatment attempts were aimed at identifying and treating diseases rather than stopping them from happening.

There is now a pressing need for a new, revived way of looking at and understanding the old concepts of human behavior and problems in living. Also called "Positive Psychology," this area concerns itself with the sunnier side of psychology, which is the population of people who are happy and optimistic and who move with confidence in whatever they do and wherever they go. Positive psychology may shed more light on why people behave in a pleasing and healthy manner and how they have developed that trait. Ironically, this new developing area of study may help us eventually find a lasting

*Allan G. Hedberg, Ph.D.*

cure for many of what we now refer to as negative psychological conditions and sick and eccentric behaviors.

Positive psychology has become the new way to redefine and readjust the existing disparity or imbalance of human life. Being a new branch of psychology, this field is still in its infant stage and is hotly contested for its veracity and advantages by both detractors and supporters. Some tend to neglect this new theory, while others vouch for its authenticity. Many individuals have not learned to believe in the concepts of joy, positive thinking, optimism, and love; others see a bright daylight in everything they do, see, and say, thus affirming the possibility of living a positive lifestyle and curing the old and common psychological disorders.

The new theories of positive psychology condemn the traditional practice of treating mental health patients merely with medication or as numbers or objects. Experts who utilize positive psychological theory have many approaches and techniques that actually have been shown to solve the many problems in living we all experience at one time or other in our life. These experts are united by the views that normal human beings possess excellent qualities and that we are still capable enough to make better choices about what we believe and do.

The salt and pepper shakers of happiness and optimism need to be on the kitchen tables of every home.

Published in Valley Health

## GOOD HABITS FOR HEALTHY LIVING

Good habits encourage others to be attracted to us and to see us as a role model for their lives. Our children, family members, neighbors and work colleagues are a few such people that may see us as their role model. How than shall we live? How do we shape our daily behavior patter so others will be drawn to us and see us as their preferred role model? Below are a few suggested behavior patterns that most of us would acknowledge as good habits.

1. **Live honestly and blamelessly**. Live peacefully with a conscience that is clear and without guilt.
2. **Practice a peaceful lifestyle**. Encourage peace by doing all you can to live peacefully so much as the power is within you to do so.
3. **Live a life of generosity.** Give generously, cheerfully and willingly both you time and your treasure; you will reap happiness.
4. **Do the best you can in each situation you undertake**. Be adequate for each task as you need not do all things perfectly.
5. **Respond to criticism with openness**. A non-defensive, open attitude, and a willingness to learn, are the best ways to confront critical people and criticism.
6. **Take time to meditate**. Reflect on your day's experiences and be sure to include your lofty thoughts of the day.
7. **Let your daily decisions reflect wisdom.** Decisions based on a good mix of emotional and rational factors yield wise outcomes.
8. **Start many projects, but finish what you start.** Do your work with diligence and determination from start to finish.

9. **Keep the faith, utmost.** Expect that something good will happen in your day. Be optimistic and hopeful.
10. **Clear the record regularly through forgiveness.** Offer and accept forgiveness for wrongs and hurts, both received and perpetrated by another person.
11. **Engage regularly in mind-stretching activities.** Learn skills and systematically expand you knowledge base on a variety of topics.
12. **Foster and strengthened social friendships.** Through regular contact and meaningful engagement with others we gain personal strength for the day and for the duties we undertake.
13. **Be a communicator in all arenas of your life.** Initiate conversation as you have opportunity and respond freely with those that engage you in dialogue.
14. **Overcome hurts and attacks with good.** Although it is difficult, our goal should be to engage in good and kindly act towards those that annoy and bother us.

While such behavior patterns may be difficult to develop and consistently life out, they are worth the effort as they bring quality to our lives and to the lives of those that identify us as their role model. Quality living is not easy, but it is rewarding and peace producing.

# FRIENDS MAKE GOOD MEDICINE

In a recent study by the California Department of Mental Health, it was found that close personal relationship may be more important to one's health and welfare than exercise or diet. Further, if one were to become ill, have surgery, or be involved in an accident, the presence of friends and their support contributes significantly to the speed and quality of the recovery process. Also, longevity of life has also been found to be associated with quality friendships. These findings led to the conclusion that friends make good medicine. There is no perfect recipe as to the ingredients that make up a healthy friendship. However, consider the following principles of a quality friendship:

1. **Friends are few.** Most people know about 75 people, out of which approximately 12 might be considered friends, 3 might be considered close friends, and only 1 might be considered an intimidate friend.
2. **Friends are prepared to sacrifice for you.** Sacrifice means the willingness to serve another, often in many small ways, rather than serving oneself.
3. **Friends takes time to know you well**. A friend is someone with whom you can be transparent, open, relaxed, and unpretentious.
4. **Friends show caring and concern at all times, unconditionally.** Even though we may not appreciate what a person does at times we can still be their friend and not forsake them.
5. **Friends remain available and are approachable during a time of need.** When in need, we desire a person who stands with us, not one who lectures us or speaks for us.

*Allan G. Hedberg, Ph.D.*

> Friendships grow on the counsel we provide each other, not the directives we impose on each other.

It is vital that we examine ourselves as to the quality of friendship we provide those around us and those within our own family. Further, we need to seek out those persons whom we consider good friends and regularly share a time of friendship together. As Abraham Lincoln stated, "For a man to have friends, he must show himself friendly." We all need to find someone towards whom we can be increasingly friendly, even amidst our busyness and out of own need for quietness. Perhaps the formation of new friends needs to be a very high priority for us.

# CONTROLLING ARGUMENTS FOR THE SAKE OF YOUR RELATIONSHIPS AND HEALTH

In his classic study of high-IQ people, psychologist Lewis M. Terman found that the factor most strongly related to marital unhappiness was argumentativeness. In fact, it was far more important than any other factor.

Arguing is generally perceived as negative and counterproductive, but some people enjoy it. They seek out conflicts, to do battle, and go for the win. For them, arguing is just another way of relating to people. Unfortunately, the relationships of such people suffer and cease to exist. And, the arguments can get out of control and become physical. If that happens, the relationship is surely at risk and dire restorative steps need to be undertaken, including individual and couples counseling. The *Pledge,* printed below, is a necessary step in correcting "out of control" arguments.

Argumentativeness has direct and profound effects on the health of both parties. Arguing adversely impacts the functioning of the heart, muscular system, hormonal system and the gastrointestinal system. Pain, digestive distress, heartburn and many other problems result.

## Steps To Control Your Argumentative Impulses

1. Argumentative people are often of above-average intelligence. So, make an intelligent self-appraisal of your own argumentative style. Observe how you deal with others and how they react to you. If you suspect that you might be overly argumentative, ask a friend to level with you.

2. Monitor what comes out of your mouth. At first you may only be able to do this after the fact, looking back on what you have said. Then try to monitor your conversation as it is going on, and, eventually monitor what you say before you say it.
3. In conversation, it is important to show with verbal and nonverbal signals that you are listening: A nod of the head, accompanied by "umhm," "I see your point," or "yeah," can help diffuse an argument. It is also helpful to periodically use the neutral phrase, "I understand."
4. If someone didn't do something that you were counting on, and you are angry, don't bring up all the other times the person has disappointed you in the past five years. Limit your anger response to what got you angry this time.
5. Compulsive arguers take the opposite point of view, whatever the subject, as a way of keeping the conversation going. They think that if they can't come up with a different or contrary point of view, there's nothing to talk about. If the conversation goes quiet because you chose to suppressed a desire to disagree, good for you. Count that period of silence as a positive point for you.
6. Develop a sense of the absurdity of life. Making your point with a joke and a smile can be 10 times more effective than zinging it with venom and a snarl.
7. Pledge to keep any and all discussions and arguments within the boundaries of control and respect for each other. Use the *Pledge* printed below to help all parties of a conflict keep themselves under control and feeling safe.

> **MY PLEDGE TO BE SELF-CONTROLLED**
>
> Dear _____,
>
> I wish to acknowledge to you my past acts of violent arguments. While I may have blamed you at the time, I was wrong to do so. I know now that I alone am responsible for my argumentative behavior, and that I alone can change it.
>
> I do not ask for your trust at this time. Just know that I want us to have the benefits of a violence and conflict-free relationship, and that I am working to change myself so that we can have it. I commit to you, with my word of honor, that my words and behavior toward you will be free of violent arguments from this time forward.
>
> _____
> Signature

In summary, the quality of our relationships and health directly results from how we treat others and how they treat us. Argumentativeness packs a hard punch to our gut and all our vital organs. Relationships live and die to the degree to which arguments and conflicts are allowed, tolerated or resolved.

# COMBATING LONELINESS IS COMBATING ILLNESS

Forming and maintaining friendships is very difficult for some people. A survey several years ago found that 1 in 6 people do not have a close friend in whom they can confide personal problems. This is especially significant when the close link between loneliness and illness is considered—single people have more illnesses and accidents than married people. Also, loneliness is often associated with depression, alcoholism and suicide.

Researchers have suggested two kinds of loneliness. One kind is related to the absence of an emotionally intimate relationship. The other kind of loneliness is associated with insufficient activities, interests and social group involvements. It can be described as social isolation. Individuals experiencing the second kind of loneliness often feel as if they don't "fit in."

When we experience the first kind of loneliness we often try to compensate by putting more energy into the relationships we already have, rather than developing new ones. This may result in a socially isolated husband or wife turning more and more to his or her spouse to fill the needs usually met by friends, work or recreational activities. Of course, this may be an impossible task for the spouse and may seriously strain the relationship. On the other hand, busy, socially active people can feel intense loneliness when they lack romantic interest or have intimate friendships. Rather than cultivating deeper relationships, however, they may become even more active and involved in work, hobbies or group activities in an attempt to keep busy and not dwell on their problems.

Everyone needs to feel unique and special to someone. We also need to feel accepted and valued as a part of a social group. To feel a kinship with others is a deep need in all of us. How can we achieve the meeting of these needs?

- Know the various kinds of relationships which need to be developed in order to deal effectively with loneliness. Otherwise you may be vulnerable and at risk for ill health.
- Decide if you need to deepen existing relationships. Try to discern and change the barriers which may be keeping emotional intimacy from developing.
- Select several activities or interests you enjoy, and join a group which promotes them. Spend some time each day engaging in the activity or learning something about it.
- Attend group meetings, classes and outings regularly. To have friends, be friendly and be a friend to many. Do something for someone; be willing to listen. Call someone to let him know you are thinking of them.

An Arabian proverb puts it this way, "A friend is one to whom one may pour out all the contents of one's heart, chaff and grain together, knowing that the gentlest of hands will sift it, keep what is worth keepings, and with a breath of kindness, blow the rest away."

# Chapter Four

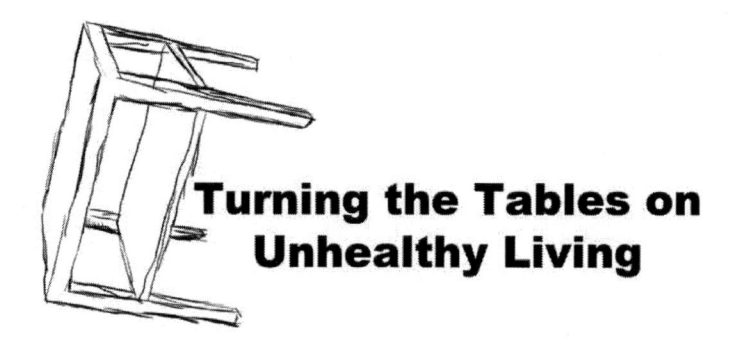

## Turning the Tables on Unhealthy Living

EVERYONE THINKS OF CHANGING THE WORLD,
BUT NO ONE THINKS OF CHANGING HIMSELF
*LEO TOLSTOY*

# TURNING THE TABLE ON STRESS

Three words describe our day and age: hurry, worry, and bury. Some have called this the race of life. Others describe us as undergoing the epidemic of hurry sickness that causes a high degree of stress. However, it is the state we are in at any given time. Many of us live lives of quiet desperation. We have all had times when we have been between a rock and a hard place. When the pressing demands of time and expectations are upon us, we need to stop and rediscover our priorities. We need to reaffirm our areas of personal strength and open our minds to learn from these experiences.

The successful executive learns very early how to handle stress well. If a company must reduce stress for the executive, it has the wrong executive. The solution is not the elimination of stress for our personal growth comes as we experience stressful events and come to terms with these events. It is not instant growth, but a painstaking process of waiting, failing, losing, struggling, and being misunderstood. As we persevere, we experience growth and maturity much like a child is able to chart his growth on the bathroom wall from year to year. Do you see progress in your ability to manage stress now in comparison to last year?

How do we turn the tables on stress and utilize it to our best advantage? How can stress become a refining tool and not the kiss of death? How do we kill stress before it kills us? Is there a balm for the stress ridden? Is there a stepping stone from distress to success? Consider the following:

1. **Approach Tasks with Affirmative Thinking.** Successful athletes, performers, and executives share the habit pattern of thinking positively on what they want to happen prior to

undertaking an assignment. It is important to develop this hopeful and positive thinking pattern about what you are going to do and what you want to happen as a result of what you do. This is sometimes referred to as "the winning feeling."

2. **Talk Out Your Worries and Fears.** Most psychologists agree that tensions are reduced by talking out your worries with a respected listener. Requesting the advice and opinions of others is not an indication of weakness, immaturity or a dependent person who cannot stand on his own two feet. Rather, it is a show of strength and that you are a person of intelligence who knows when to ask questions and receive assistance.

3. **Respond to the Needs of Others**. When distressed, we tend to concentrate on ourselves and on our own situation. This indwelling only heightens the strong emotions of stress, anger, frustration, resentment, and sorrow. Seek out ways to respond to the needs of others. Be aware of those around you. This reduces the concentration on oneself and helps us view our own situation in a more positive light.

4. **Undertake One Thing at a Time.** It is defeating to attempt to tackle all your problems at once. For people under normal tension, an ordinary work load can sometimes seem unbearable. It is important to remember that it is a temporary condition and that you can work your way out of it by taking one problem at a time. Take a few of the most urgent tasks or the task that you are likely to succeed in resolving, and pitch into them, setting aside the other tasks until later. Give thought to a priority list when undertaking a series of tasks to be accomplished. Establishing priorities can be invaluable strategy whenever pressured builds up on all sides.

5. **Delegate to Others.** Tackling all the tasks and responsibilities that come to you in the course of our day can be folly and an exercise in being overwhelmed. Stress can be moderated through delegation of tasks and authority. Wise delegation first requires the selection of colleagues who are known for their honesty, dependability, mature judgment, and demonstrated experience in problem solving. Successful

executives surround themselves with successful colleagues who can be called upon in a time of need to share their concerns and responsibilities with them. Stop the destructive thinking that you can do it all, that no one can do it as well as you, that no one cares as much as you, or that no one else understands like you do. Train others to care, understand and take action, and let them do so.

6. **Avoid Self Medication.** It is easy to become part of a vicious cycle of stress leading to the consumption of anything from anti-acids to tranquilizers and then the increase of further stress and so on. No prescription, alcohol, drugs—or any mixture of any of these can take on the battle of banishing those stressful events in your life. Self-medication is like a Mardi Gras mask; it does not help you to adjust to the stress itself. Most of these self inflicted measures become habit forming. The ability to handle stress is learned and comes from within you, not from external things we ingest for temporary relief. Look not for an external ways to spell RELIEF, but develop the ability to mold stress into a valuable asset of your personality and character. This requires total thought and adaptability. A dulled mind and clumsy coordination only gives stress the upper hand and perpetuates a vicious cycle.

*Allan G. Hedberg, Ph.D.*

---

**Prevention of Stress**

1. Recognize and define what causes stress.
2. Plan for forthcoming major changes and high-stress projects.
3. Learn to compromise and live with imperfections in yourself and others.
4. Maintain a strong support group of friends and family members.
5. Avoid self-medication.
6. Maintain a good self-image and accept that which cannot be changed.
7. Be self-expressive and able to self-disclose.
8. Delegate and share responsibilities.
9. Limit projects to a manageable number.
10. Do what is right; ethically, legally, and morally.

---

It is vital to clarify and claim a code of life, to know how to live. It might be suggested that a port of destination and a purpose for living be identified and claimed. A port of destination might be to acquire as much good will and as many friends as possible. This may lead to the feelings of acceptance, support and wellness. What is your port of destination? Where does all your hurry and worry lead you? By turning stress into a positive force in our lives, we make known to all that we are headed in the right direction and that our next port of call is one to which we will devote our energy, efforts, and determination. Stress is a cruel taskmaster, take charge of the stressful situation, adjust to its challenge, and turn the tables on stress.

# TURNING THE TABLE ON DEPRESSION

Next to anxiety, depression is the most frequently encountered psychological problem found among Americans. Approximately, 15% of the population experiences depression at some time in their life. Typical self-defeating thoughts of people who are depressed are statements such as, "I'm such a lousy secretary." "Nothing I ever do turns out right." "I just can't get myself motivated." "Maybe I should dissolve my marriage."

Self-defeating thoughts similar to these contribute to the change in the way a person comes to act and think about himself. Negative changes in one's thinking, feeling, and behaving are a key feature in depression. Lifestyle changes generally come about gradually, but can occur immediately following a major traumatic event, such as the death of a spouse or child. Other major life changes that often create depression might be a business reversal, job termination, financial setback, chronic criticism of one's work, and a series of business and personal decisions that turned sour.

Instead of seeking pleasure and dealing with the depressing issues facing a person, the depressed individual tends to avoid others, and often involves himself in elaborate schemes of withdrawal and escapism. Instead of caring for himself, he neglects himself and his appearance. His instinct to survive and succeed may give way to a desire to end life. The drive to achieve goals may be replaced by passivity and defeatism.

The most obvious and typical signs of depression are seen in the moods of sadness, gloom, loneliness, and apathy. Sleeping problems, withdrawal, constant tiredness, pain, the loss of appetite and weight are other signs of depression. Negative self reference

*Allan G. Hedberg, Ph.D.*

statements, the feeling of helplessness, blaming one's self for faults and shortcomings, being pessimistic, trouble making decisions, and the loss of interests are additional symptoms of depression.

Further, depression has been associated with increased risk of diabetes, hypertension, and cardiovascular disease. A number of studies have assessed the association between depression and the risk of stroke morbidity and mortality, suggesting that depression could be a modifiable risk factor for stroke. Ongoing research on this topic at the Harvard School of Public Health seems to demonstrate that depression is prospectively associated with a significantly increased risk of developing a stroke. An association was found between depression and strokes. The reason this topic is of great interest is due to the significant economic and physical losses and the permanent disability often associated with a stroke.

How does one turn the tables on depression? How do we break the vicious cycle of defeatism, withdrawal, passivity, detachment, and feelings of helplessness? First, dispel the myths of depression. False beliefs must be corrected and the problem of depression approached in a forthright manner. Below are the key myths that one must challenge and dispel.

# MYTHS ABOUT DEPRESSION

The following myths of depression need to be addressed with all or most depressed persons as the beginning of their healing process. People with depression express relief when the myths they consider to be true are confronted and dispelled.

MYTH 1—People who become depressed have weak characters.
*It is not a character issue, but an emotional and situational issue.*

MYTH 2—Depression is shared equally by both sexes.
*It is more often seen in women.*

MYTH 3—Depression is always caused by emotional distress.
*No, it is more often situational in nature, but affects one's emotions.*

MYTH 4—Depression is unpleasant, but it cannot make you physically sick.
*It is not uncommon for depressed people to manifest illness and sickness.*

MYTH 5—Your age has nothing to do with your likelihood of becoming depressed.
*More often seen in older people, but affects all ages.*

MYTH 6—Depression does not destroy your desire for sexual romance.
*Sexual desire and performance are greatly affected by depression.*

MYTH 7—A person with depression will always feel better in time, even without therapy or medication.
*While time has healing affects, depression can linger without treatment.*

MYTH 8—Treatment of depression inevitably means years of psychotherapy.

*It is not uncommon for treatment to be brief, although it may open other areas on which to focus during therapy and extend it accordingly.*

MYTH 9—The psychological triggers for a period of depression are always obvious.
*More often than not, the triggering event(s) may be obscure and covert.*

MYTH 10—You can be treated effectively for depression by the use of medication alone.
*The most effective therapy is psychotherapy and medication used together.*

MYTH 11—You can always help a person with depression with some old fashioned pep talks, especially when using some well known quotations.
*This strategy has been found to make matters worse, not better.*

MYTH 12—An episode of depression is sure to leave scars.
*No, while it may be a memory, it may yield more benefits than harm.*

MYTH 13—Depression will always return in time if you have had one episode of depression.
*No, most people learn better coping skills from the experience and are better at preventing depression from recurring.*

What positive changes need to take place? A series of psychological research studies have shown that depression can be prevented or significantly altered if a series of constructive actions are undertaken. These include the following:

1. **Engage in mastery and measurable activities.** Each day plan a few activities that involve some mastery of the situation and some activities that will bring you pleasure. At the end of each day, take inventory to assure yourself that you, in fact, have engaged in both types of activities during that day. Start off with activities which are easy and simple and then progress to those which are more difficult and complex.

2. **Increase the rewards derived from daily living.** Depressed people tend not to reward themselves or accept the rewards expressed to them by others. It is important to allow yourself to be praised, complimented and affirmed by others and to express these kinds of statements to yourself upon behaving in a manner which is desirable and productive.
3. **Engage in assertive communication patterns.** Rather than being passive and withdrawn, express your feelings desires, and preferences to others so that they better understand you and can respond to your needs in a more satisfying manner. There are times to say "no" and there are times to say "yes." There are times to ask for help and times to turn down the suggestions and help of others when it is not desired or appropriate. Basically, we need to learn how to get from others what we need and want. We need to learn how to limit and control the degree to which other people overpower and take control.
4. **Correct irrational thinking patterns.** Negative thinking and expectations of the future may include irrational thoughts. What a person thinks about certainly affects how he feels at the time. For example, depressed people feel sad and lonely because they erroneously think of themselves as being inadequate and deserted. Do not focus on the depressed mood, but rather change your errors in thinking. Be optimistic, realistic, and rational in thinking. Ask others to tell you how your thinking is irrational and what it would take to correct it.
5. **Develop problem solving skills.** If a particular task seems complex and burdensome, try writing down the steps that need to be undertaken to accomplish the task. Then, undertake one step at a time. Proceed from the known to the unknown, and from the simple to the complex. Accept help from others when needed.
6. **Increase social involvement.** Rather than withdraw and isolate, seek out other people, particularly supportive people. It is not proper to avoid all people, but only people who add to your depression. Be around and bring into your life those people who increase your stimulation and feelings

of wellness. With positively oriented persons, engage in social activities which add to your feelings of pleasure and happiness.
7. **Think in a futuristic and positive manner.** Negative thinking adds to the depression, whereas a positive outlook about the future is anti-depressing. With the help of others, one can retrain thinking patterns in 10 weeks. For example, what do you want more of in the future? What goals would you like to see achieved? It is not a quick fix, to be sure, but a good outcome when positive thinking rules the day.

In summary, depression is a major emotional state that affects about 15 percent of the general population at some time in their adult life. Depression can be prevented and altered once it occurs. It is a direct result of one's life experiences and one's life style.

Psychotherapy may be helpful to find ways to deal more effectively with real day-to-day problems in living. It is designed to help you learn to respond with less depression and misery when you encounter difficulties in the future. Further, it is conducted to identify and correct unrealistic beliefs and thinking patterns. It is not a matter of coping with depression, but changing it. Take responsibility to turn the tables on depression.

# TURNING THE TABLE ON BURNOUT

BURNOUT. For many, this word is associated with gray ashes, dying embers, or a final flickering flame. Others may think of a dying battery or an empty teapot. Remember when you were all fired up about your involvement with other people? You were excited, full of energy, dedicated, committed and willing to give beyond what seemed reasonable for the sake of others. Over time, you may have given, given, and given until finally there is nothing left to give anymore. Without any energy and motivational replacement, burnout occurs.

Burnout is defined as a syndrome of emotional exhaustion, de-personalization, and the feeling of reduced personal accomplishment that primarily occurs among individuals who do "people work" in the form of service. Chronic emotional strain is a natural experience when dealing extensively and regularly with troubled persons. Although it is a type of job stress, it is particularly the stress that arises from the social or helping interaction between a helper and a recipient.

Burnout is reflected on the state of one's health. Burnout is associated with depression post trauma stress systems, chronic pain, insomnia, anxiety, panic attacks, chest pain, headaches and gastrointestinal distress, to name a few health-related problems.

## Am I Experiencing Burnout?

The following feelings, attitudes, and expressed reflections are often associated with people who are burnt out:

- "It's not that I don't want to help, but I just can't."
- "I am becoming calloused toward people."
- "It's painful to admit, but maybe I'm just not cut out for this work."
- "I could care less."
- "Do I have to go to work today?"
- "I'm having no influence on the lives of people through my work anymore."

## Am I Among The Vulnerable?

Research and burnout identifies a general lifestyle among those most vulnerable to burnout. You are vulnerable if you have:

- Idealistic and over-committed expectations.
- Rigid and high standards
- Intense commitment to social change.
- A desire to avoid conflict and satisfy everybody.
- Constant demands to meet the needs of the poor, dying, sick and hurting.
- Role confusion and unclear purpose.
- Failed to protect your personal boundaries for rest, relationships and relaxation.

Some careers that are most vulnerable to the burnout experience include teachers, ministers, counselors, health care providers, social service administrators and a variety of allied health professionals.

## Is It Me Or My Job?

It's both. While many live a high stress lifestyle and do not possess the personality traits which give strength, stamina and balance, psychologists generally find that burnout occurs in the high stress job settings. The common denominator is overload—emotional and/or physical. When feeling overloaded, there is a tendency to pull back psychologically and become less involved in the lives of others, especially with those who seek our services. Feeling overwhelmed, we tend to look for ways out of the situation and withdraw. We cry out for a new job description, a redefinition of responsibilities and tasks. We take time off and often find a pattern of illness occurring.

Further, job burnout occurs when we feel out of control, helpless and when our destiny is in the hands of an unkind superior, rigid rules, and unfair policies. Office traditions and sundry red tape can be stress producing also. Administrative inconveniences and over-reach are like water on a burning flame.

It often appears that if the clients, patients, students or recipients of services rendered don't get you, co-workers surely will. In many work settings, the lack of rapport among staff places undue strain on the worker and saps energy. Distrust, competition, jealousies, in-fighting, back-biting and similar petty relationships constitute the battle of the burnout day after day after day. We often call it a morale problem.

## From Whence Cometh My Help?

There are answers, but they come hard. They come from personal reflection, reorganization of lifestyle, assertive and confrontive approaches to other people, and even from creative and constructive change in the work place. Here are a few ideas to get you started:

- Re-examine your goals and make them more realistic. After all, you now know more about what is possible in the work place than when you first took the job.
- Do the same thing differently by changing routine, scheduling, sequence, and even bending the rules and procedures.
- Taking care of "Number One" is an essential prerequisite for taking care of others. Don't give your personal needs and interests the lowest priority of your time and involvements. Take time for yourself. Renew yourself daily.
- Diversify your involvements. Have clear boundaries between your job and your home. At some point, you must leave your

*Allan G. Hedberg, Ph.D.*

work setting psychologically as well as physically. Similarly, diversify your friendships and your associations. Isolation adds to burnout. Do not underestimate the power of companionship and social support. In your leisure time, be sure to include people who have nothing to do with your line of work. They add a different perspective to your thinking.
- Change jobs or careers. Changes can be for the better, but there is no guaranteed success. A well-planned change can be a positive step in personal growth. It should be considered a crucial step in the process of taking stock of yourself in order to take better care of yourself.
- When you find yourself just trying to cope with the work environment, take steps to change it. Do what you can to make the job and the setting less stressful and boring. Associate with different people than is usually the case. Arrange for help and be available to help others so that the work gets accomplished more easily.

In summary, the basic message about burnout is to balanced giving to others and giving to yourself. Making yourself strong, knowledgeable, and assertive makes you a better provider for those in need. You may also be a healthier colleague for those with whom you work. As a result, those whom you serve will benefit and enjoy a healthy relationship with you. Maintain a sense of personal autonomy and control over what you do for others and allow others to impose upon you. Take stock of your life now so that burnt out is not your epitaph. Rather, recapture the zeal and excitement which you brought to your job originally. It is possible to care for others without paying the high cost of burnout.

# THE TRAUMA CONUNDRUM

Bad things happen to good people; bad things happen to innocent people and unsuspecting people. Bad things can be traumatic, but not necessarily. To be sure, there are many bad experiences in life which upset us, distress us, or hurt us, but not to the level of a trauma. The term trauma is reserved to describe those events which go beyond the pale of human experience of everyday life, and pose a threat to our health, safety, and our life. At least 2% of the population has been diagnosed with a post trauma stress disorder due to some traumatic event or series of events.

Within the mental health professions, the recognized diagnostic criteria for a traumatic event are fairly clear. A person has been exposed to a traumatic event in which both of the following were present:

1. The person experienced, witnessed, or was confronted with an event or series of events that involved actual or threatened death or serious injury, or a threat to the physical integrity of self or others.
2. The person's response involved intense fear, helplessness, or horror.

## Trauma and Abuses

Traumas come in many forms of life-threatening and life-changing events. They produce lingering effects on the way one thinks, feels, perceives, remembers, make decisions, relates interpersonally and even the quality of sleep.

*Allan G. Hedberg, Ph.D.*

For the majority of us, the effects of a traumatic event linger for 6 to 9 months with the aid of medical and psychological treatment. Should the person refuse treatment or treatment is not available, the lingering effects could be 6 to 18 months or more in duration.

Of course, there are reasons why a traumatized person would choose not to benefit from the array of community based treatment approaches that are available. Some choose not to benefit because of their strong belief in self-help, while others are disingenuous and attempt to gain certain financial or sympathetic advantages by prolonging or heightening the trauma experience and the associated injuries.

Unfortunately, a post-trauma stress disorder has also been abused. For example, there are times when the post-trauma stress disorder diagnosis is used inappropriately as the event and injuries do not meet the criteria set forth by the profession. There are those that utilize the diagnosis as an excuse to remain in the mode of a victim. And there are those that malinger and prolong their recovery to obtain financial benefit, jockey for legal advantage in a lawsuit or justify not returning to an unpleasant employment situation.

## Profiles of Trauma

The trauma experience is very individualized. That is, trauma to one person may not be trauma to another. We all bring our own personal experiences to the traumatizing event. Our perception and reaction to the trauma event is strongly influenced by our personality traits, level of social support, faith and values, preparedness, arousal threshold, cognitive functioning, and prior similar experiences. Consider a few examples.

Mary, who had never been involved in a prior automobile accident or major injury, perceived her accident much more traumatically than others may have perceived it. Others did not believe her incident was that traumatizing. She recovered completely after 4 months of therapy.

Joel, who survived a 50 foot fall from a construction scaffold, felt severely traumatized for over a year and never did overcome his fear of heights. He avoided the offer of therapy.

Martina maintained a fear of flying for fifteen years after her airplane flight out of Fresno, CA ran into severe turbulence and had to undertake an emergency landing. She denied the referral to a therapist.

Raul double locks and double checks his door every night since he learned of the traumatic home invasion of his house was perpetrated by a local gang, all armed with guns. Raul started therapy years after the event, but was partially helped, nonetheless.

As a psychotherapist, I find that trauma cases come with intense urgency. They cover a wide variety of life-threatening and life-changing events. Those that seek psychotherapy besides medical treatment recover more quickly and more fully.

## Can We Prepare For A Trauma?

The answer is both yes and no. Trauma generally comes at an unexpected time and in an unexpected manner. Usually, our attention and energies are focused at the time on other events and problems in life. In other words, they generally catch us unaware. Lack of prepared readiness is one reason why some people do not recover well from a trauma event.

On the other hand, knowing that trauma is real and does enter the life of at least 2% of the population, pre-trauma preparation is wise and recommended. For example, here are some things to do to ready oneself:

1. Read about the traumatic stressful event in the lives of people. Learn how they handled them and recovered from them.

2. When appropriate, discuss with people their trauma experience and imagine how you would have handled the event had that trauma happened to you.
3. Learn the skills that are necessary to overcome trauma, such as learning how to relax, how to interpret events as opportunities for growth rather than being a demoralized victim, and learning the positive meaning of mottos, such as, "Where there is no pain, there is no gain."
4. Belong to a positive and healthy social and faith affirming social network.

## Respond To Trauma, Don't React

When a trauma experience enters your life, think through a systematic organized response that will likely lead to recovery. Don't just react as a reaction is merely an emotional knee jerk promise to change or get help, but without the intent to follow through. Little systematic long-term benefit results when the knee jerk reaction pattern is followed.

Trauma recovery depends on a systematic pattern of rethinking the trauma, rebuilding the body, reorganizing one's lifestyle and reaffirming one's faith and values. Consider the following steps:

1. Immediately seek medical and psychological professional assistance.
2. Sleep 8 to 10 hours a night with a 1-hour daytime power nap.
3. Use an antidepressant to assist in regulating the emotions associated with any losses and prevents lingering debilitating emotions from developing.
4. Walk and talk about the trauma event with those from your support network, and particularly to those professionally trained and experienced in treating trauma.
5. Engage in light exercise, as appropriate, to help distribute the flow of adrenalin that is naturally produced in excess at the time of a trauma and for a short period of time thereafter.

6. Consider how forgiveness for trauma resolution is relevant in your case.

## Friends Make Good Medicine

There are simple things that friends can do to help. Positive help comes in the form supporting words, a reassuring touch, progressive actions and a caring attitude. Here are some specifics:

1. Send a letter or card expressing support and ongoing interest.
2. Avoid clichés and easy phrases and mottos. Be sincere.
3. Keep in contact and follow through with what you say or promise.
4. Offer to help with practical day-to-day matters such as meals, shopping, providing care for the children and the routine household chores.
5. Encourage other people to visit and guide them in how they might best help.
6. Listen well and do more listening than talking.
7. Do not probe or force discussion about the details of the trauma. Let the details freely emerge as the person is ready to talk.
8. Don't talk about trivial matters with the traumatized person or family members, rather be serious and respectful.
9. Encourage easy activity and exposure as appropriate to outside light and fresh air.
10. Beware that recovery comes slowly and progresses systematically.

## Trauma in Summation

Trauma changes us. In an instant we become a different person. We now view the world and ourselves most differently. While we all choose to react or respond to trauma differently, our preparedness and our assertive entry into a treatment format will largely determine

*Allan G. Hedberg, Ph.D.*

if we recover or fall into a victim role. Secondary motivations, our faith and values and our personality traits also contribute to the way and degree we recover for a trauma.

Trauma is a huge experience to process. But the human passion and commitment to health and wellness is bigger. While defeat and loss is possible at the time of a life-changing event, recovery and personal growth do result from an intentional pursuit through treatment.

Published in the Valley Health Magazine, December/January, 2007

# THE PAIN OF DISCOURAGEMENT: IS THERE A WAY OUT?

Discouragement is a part of the human experience. For some, it comes into our lives momentarily and periodically. For others, it is a 24-hour marathon challenge in coping and survival. We often wonder if darkness will ever break into dawn. Feelings of helplessness and hopelessness are not uncommon. Headaches, chills, depression, fatigue, and muscular tightness are also fairly common manifestations of discouragement.

The pale of discouragement demands our understanding and the creation of strategies for change, whether we experience it for brief periods of time or live with it daily. We all have our story to relate, even though it is painful to tell. Unfortunately, we tend to go silent, isolate and withdraw when discouraged. That can make matters worse.

Discouragement can be best understood in the dialogue that took place between a western cowboy and two buffalos. The story unfolded in the western plains, "out where the buffalo roam, and the deer and the antelope play." We all remember the song very well. One day, a cowboy rode up to two buffaloes standing and contemplating the course of their day. The cowboy remarked to the buffaloes, "You guys are pitiful. Your coat is mangy, dirty, and unkempt. You smell. You stand there hunched over, looking down at the ground. Your long face is pitiful. You should feel ashamed of yourselves." At that point, the cowboy rode off and left the buffaloes standing there. Reflecting on what they had just heard, one buffalo said to the other, "We have just heard the discouraging word."

For many of us, the above story repeats itself as part of our daily experience. We live with and relate to people who are critical, negative and sarcastic. Put down words are all too frequently expressed. They are devastating, indeed.

To cope with discouragement, it is necessary to understand the sources of discouragement in our life. We are then in a better position to learn the skills of managing it's impact effectively.

## Components of Discouragement

1. Facing an overwhelming task.
2. Laboring under demanding and unrealistic expectations.
3. Anticipating strong opposition from unexpected persons.
4. Progressing in a task in a slow and microscopic manner.

## Self Management Strategies

Discouragement acts like a stinger. It hits and hurts. It may immobilize us for a brief time, but has the potential to become a way of life. Repeated hits are worse. We can choose to endure, avoid, deny, and just ride out the circumstances. Or, we can assertively react to bring about change in the circumstances and in our ability and skill to manage such experiences effectively. Consider the following managing strategies for turning the tables on discouragement:

1. Expect opposition, even from friends.
2. Strike a positive ratio between planning and action; more planning than action.
3. Keep your eye on the goal, a goal that is bigger than yourself.
4. Utilize motivating reminders, mottos, slogans, and stories.
5. Build your network of social support and stick together.
6. Establish a system to guard yourself from additional assault.
7. Learn confrontive, assertive communication skills.

Finally, become a person of encouragement. Live your life so that others draw strength from you and do not lose strength. As you engage in actions of encouragement, you will be less susceptible to the acts and words of discouragement from others. As you confront the painful situations of discouragement, you will start feeling better and stronger. Health factors will improve. It is all about getting up one more time than falling down. It is also disregarding the words of negative people and turning towards the positive people in your life.

# THE EIGHT R's OF ANXIETY MANAGEMENT

Anxiety is one of the strongest, most pervasive and life-interfering emotions common to our daily living experience. Anxiety prevents us from entering into a wide variety of social situations and relationships. Anxiety is the basis of a host of physical ailments, fatigue and other forms of self-defeating behavior. Below are eight well-accepted tools for the management of anxiety. These tools should be utilized over a 90-day time period for best results to occur. They can be used as part of a professional treatment program.

**Anti-Anxiety Actions**

1. **Recognize anxiety feelings.** Since one is not always anxious it is important to identify the onset and build-up of anxiety feelings so that corrective action can be taken early rather than waiting until the feelings become overwhelming. Anxiety is generally identified with the increase of apprehensiveness, worry, agitation, arousal and a feeling of readiness to "fight or flight." These feelings occur over time and generally increase in intensity if not addressed and corrected.
2. **Research the triggering events.** Anxiety is always associated with certain specific events which trigger adrenalin flow and fear. These are usually identifiable. Such triggers might precede the feelings of anxiety by minutes, hours or days. The stimulus-response linkage is essential to identify if anxiety is to be controlled and managed.
3. **Reframe the anxiety situation.** We often experience anxiety because we over interpret what might happen to us. Be careful not to catastrophize your view of the situation.

Do not see it as a plot against you by anyone. Rather, see the situation as something about which to be cautious and careful, but not anxious or fearful. Also, even anxious experiences can promote laughter. See the growth potential that may be present.

4. **Relaxation training is essential.** When a person is anxious, the body responds with increased tension throughout the muscle system and there is a heightened feeling of nervousness. The glands are all secreting their various hormones. This gives a sense of unrest and arousal. The opposite response is one of relaxation and calmness. The muscles can be trained to let go so that a state of calm and ease prevails. The muscle system is like a rubber band that one can tighten or let go.

5. **Re-orient your perception.** During times of anxiety, one's perception can be distracted away from the anxiety situation to something more neutral or relaxing. Play relaxing music. Be around people who create and atmosphere of relaxation. Look away. Do not pay attention to the feelings of the body but, rather, to a neutral stimulus present in the environment at the time.

6. **Reduce avoidance behavior.** There is a strong tendency to try to escape from, and avoid, any situation that creates feelings of anxiety and unrest. We never get over anxiety in that manner. It is important to stay in the situation. Use the relaxation response, re-orient your perception, re-frame the situation and learn to deal with the fear situation directly. Learn that you can handle it. Learn that it is not as dangerous as you thought. Once you learn that the anxiety can be reduced while still in the situation or anticipating the situation, you are on the main road to recovery.

7. **Repeat approach behavior.** While one should not avoid anxiety-provoking situations, one also needs to learn how to approach those situations safely and comfortably. It is best to make gradual steps in approaching the situation that is causing the anxiety. Start out taking one step that is easy and comfortable and then gradually increase it while maintaining relaxation and a feeling of calm. Back up a little

if the anxiety increases. Then go forward again. Approaching the fear situation should be handled in gradual, incremental steps.
8. **Engage in an act of quieting the mind and body.** When stress is encountered and distress feelings are evident, take a few moments and engage in the *Quieting Response Exercise* as printed below. Do it several times daily.

---

### QUIETING RESPONSE EXERCISE

Whenever you encounter a stressful situation and wish to relax check your breathing. If it is shallow, indicating tension, smile and say to yourself, "What a stupid thing to do to my body." Next, take a slow, easy, deep breath into a count of five. Hold and let go to a slow, easy, deep count of five. Now take another easy breath. As you exhale to an easy slow count of five, let your body go totally limp. Drop your jaw and let it go completely limp. Let your lips go limp. Imagine feelings of warmth and heaviness flowing from your neck down to your toes at about the same time as you exhale and let all the breath out. Now, enjoy the state of relaxation. After a minute or two, carry on your normal activity.

---

Consistently taking the above steps can lead to better health and a greater sense of ease and control over one's life. The hassles and stresses that life brings our way certainly will not disappear. Anyone can learn to respond to life's stresses in a confident and relaxed manner.

# TEMPERS CAN BE TEMPERED

Being on the end of someone's temper blowout is no picnic. A person with a short fuse and/or a bad temper is to be avoided. Such individuals have few friends and often no close friends. Tempers out of control keep others at bay. They often are the basis of a relationship terminating, as in a divorce or friends going separate ways.

A temper episode is a fully physical event. A red face and ears may be noted. The voice will vary in tone and intensity. The face muscles tighten. The jaw also tightens. One may sweat and become clammy. Hand and body tremors are notable. Tempering the temper and the related physical reaction patterns is no easy task. Self-control needs to be learned and can be learned.

A person with chronic and regular temper episodes places himself at risk for a variety of serious health related problems. A temper does not only have ill-effects on others, but on oneself also. Here is a list of some known health problems directly related to a lifestyle of a bad temper.

## Temper and Health Problems

- **Increased risk for heart related disorders.** Heart disease, heart attacks, elevated blood pressure are the most frequent corollaries of anger and temper tantrums.
- **Increased risk of gastrointestinal problems.** Digestive problems, heart burn, cramps, and an irritable bowel syndrome may well result from a lifestyle of temper tantrums.

- **Increased risk for headaches and jaw aches.** Headaches may originate from the blood pressure elevating, the facial and neck muscles tensing and from clenching the teeth and tightening the jaw muscles.
- **Increased risk for ulcers.** Temper may set the normal digestive process out of whack. A tense stomach muscle can create bleeding ulcers and cramping.
- **Increased risk for stroke.** Temper driven strokes can be fatal or debilitating a major portion of the body and leave a person without mobility.
- **Increased risk for low grade chronic illness.** Tempers uncontrolled can be associated with chronic colds, repeated sickness, and tiredness.

## How to Temper Your Tensions

1. **Talk it out.** Telling your troubles to a friend often puts your problems in a clearer light, makes them seem less desperate.
2. **Give in occasionally, even when you know you are right.** You do not have to win every point.
3. **Take one thing at a time.** When there is just too much to do, agonizing won't accomplish a thing. But doing as much as possible will work wonders sometimes.
4. **Shun the superman urge.** Shooting for perfection is an invitation for failure.
5. **Go easy with criticism.** Expecting too much of others is also an invitation to disappointment and frustration.
6. **Make yourself available.** Withdrawing from people or problems for an extended period of time generally compounds anxiety and frustration rather than allaying it.
7. **Schedule your recreation.** With a set routine of relaxation, tensions never get a chance to build up to the point where they become a threat to mental health.
8. **Figure out what you're really angry about.** Are you upset at the current situation, or is your discontent a carryover from previous events?

9. **Excuse yourself for a few minutes if possible.** Walking away from a volatile situation gives you a chance to collect yourself and measure your reaction.
10. **Accept that some things are beyond your control.** Picking ones battle is critical in all relationships. Address what can be controlled and changed. Let other things go for the time being.

Selecting from the action steps above should allow anyone to gain a fairly good control of their emotions. One's temper need not be out of control. It does take a systematic approach to temper control to establish positive relationships and succeed in marriage, employment, friendships and leadership. Health factors are also closely aligned with emotions control. The heart is the primary organ at risk. Protect your heart by learning to control the temper. Save your relationships by using the pledge statement below.

---

**COMMITMENT TO A VIOLENCE-FREE RELATIONSHIP**

Dear _____,

    I wish to acknowledge to you my past acts of violence. While I may have blamed you at the time, I was wrong to do so. I know now that I alone am responsible for my behavior, and that I alone can change it.

    I do not ask for your trust at this time. Just know that I want us to have the benefits of a violence-free relationship, and that I am working to change myself so that we can have them. I commit to you, with my word of honor, that my words and behavior toward you will be violence-free from this time forward.

_____
Signature

# DISTINCTIVES OF THE TYPE A PERSONALITY

Over thirty years ago, two cardiologists, Dr. Meyer Friedman and Ray Rosenman, began to study the non-medical risk factors associated with the onset of a heart attack. Their observations were profound and opened up an area of study that has caught the attention of the medical and psychological community. Lifestyle and heart functioning were found to be directly related.

What the doctors noticed was the fact that their patients were known to be uncommonly ambitious, striving, competitive, hard-driving, and hurried. They labeled such persons as Type A and contrasted them with those that were more relaxed. They labeled such individuals as Type B.

A subsequent study of over 3,000 healthy California men took physicals, and answered questions specifically regarding their ambitions, job involvements, urgency about time, and their need for achievement, among other areas of interest.

The results seemed to confirm their theory of the Type A personality. Over the next eight to nine years, those that were labeled Type A were more than twice as likely to suffer heart attacks as those labeled Type B, even when other factors like cholesterol levels and smoking were controlled. Subsequent studies have supported the distinction between Type A and Type B personalities. The major identifying components of a Type A personality have consistently been identified as follows:

1. A competitive, hard-driving way of life.

2. A sense of time urgency that combines speed, patience, and obsessive concern with doing more and more in less and less time.
3. Excessive involvement in one's job.

Competitive drive and impatience places a person at risk. It is now generally thought that Type A personalities must maintain a high drive and rapid pace in order to assert personal control and gain mastery over their environment. This has been shown in many subsequent research studies.

The research work by another psychologist, Dr. Charles Spielberger, identified seven distinctive qualities of the Type A personality. They are:

1. Potential for hostility.
2. Gets angry more than once a week.
3. Anger directed outward rather than towards oneself.
4. Irritability at having to wait in lines.
5. Competitiveness in games with peers.
6. Explosive modulation is lacking
7. Vigorous responses to interview questions.

Anger seemed to be the common thread that wove itself through the seven deadly behavior patterns noted above. Hostility, irritability, impatience, explosive behavior and other symptoms added up to the plain and fancy version of being a hot head. Unresolved anger and hostility seems to be the key elements contributing to heart trouble. Further, it does not seem to matter whether the anger is expressed or held in check. What would seem to be important is the frequency with which intense anger and rage are experienced. That is, venting rage does not reduce its ill effects. Concealing it does not dilute the rage nor the ill-effects of anger on the body.

The words of the Chinese proverb, "The fire you kindle for your enemy often burns you more than him" are informative. We now have urgent and personal reasons to learn to control the most self-centered and destructive of all emotions, anger.

*Allan G. Hedberg, Ph.D.*

Type B individuals are known for their slower and softer approach with others. They are low keyed and deliberate in their manner. While they are productive, they approach tasks and jobs calmer and with less feeling of distress. Anger is much less likely to be revealed or acted out on others. Type B people are generally low in anger and distress. They are more inclusive of others and take their time to undertake an action plan. Overall, Type B individuals are easy to be around and work with on a daily assignment. Kindness and consideration characterizes them. Type B behavior can be learned and appreciated. Try it!

# COPING WELL WITH PAIN, ILLNESS AND DISABILITY

Physical pain, impairment, or disability comes in various forms. It may result from injury, disease, unrelenting stress, illness or surgery. For most people, pain, reduced range of motion and dysfunctional living may occur temporarily. For others, such conditions linger and disrupt almost every aspect of their lifestyle. The mere passage of time does not bring about healing and recovery. In such cases, an aggressive, persistent and graduated sequence of activities may prove to be restorative.

Below are guidelines that have been found to be helpful in coping effectively with chronic states of disability.

1. **Learn to relax.** Relax for at least 20 minutes a day. Research has shown that relaxation can lead to better decision-making, clearer thinking, and increased energy. Use progressive relaxation, yoga, biofeedback, exercise, catnaps, and/or meditation.
2. **Learn when to take an emotional breather.** When pressure begins to build and become intense, take some time out. Go for a walk, read a book, see a movie—anything that will help you relax just when you need it. You may gain some distance from your problem and with it, some perspective.
3. **Build up physical strength.** Exercise diverts from problem-oriented thinking and increases energy and strength. According to Dr. Donald Rockwell, aerobic exercise can "lower your thermostat" to its normal level. Make daily use of systematic walking opportunities.
4. **Express anger appropriately.** When you are angry, do not hold it to yourself and buy an ulcer with silence. Learn to

express yourself with consideration, but be sure to speak up. Denying anger may lead to chronic, serious physical and emotional problems.
5. **Make your home your castle.** Everything outside your front door may be outside of your control, but make sure your home is comfortable and organized. A haven when you really need one is the essence of a home for those in distress.
6. **Set priorities.** You cannot do everything and you certainly cannot do everything well. Rather than be frantic, make a list of things you must do, in their order of importance. Set out to do them systematically, without pressure. Start with an easy task.
7. **Rely not on tranquilizers and other drugs.** Drugs are not a cure for anxiety, pain or discomfort. At best, they may be a crutch or support while you confront underlying problems through other methods, such as psychotherapy. Drugs may create other problems. Research has shown that anti-anxiety medications, such as Valium and Ativan, may lower concentration, impair memory, decrease reading skills and increase the difficulty of manual tasks. One study revealed that a similar drug, Librium, may actually increase tension and produce feelings of aggression. Remember alcohol is a highly addictive drug, as is cigarette smoking and a host of allergy drugs.
8. **Talk out your problems.** Problems seem much worse when you keep them to yourself. Talking to a spouse or a trusted friend can lighten your load and make anxieties fade. These confidants may give you a different perspective on worries. Enlisting support from friends and/or a respected professional may be helpful to you.
9. **Control worry behavior.** Try to keep your worries in perspective. Dean Williams R. Inge said worry is "interest paid on trouble before it is due." Take action to replace or over-ride worry.
10. **Learn self talk to control pain and stress.** The following series of statements can be helpful to control pain and stress. Learn them by memory and repeat them often throughout the day.

> **PAIN CONTROL STATEMENTS**
>
> - I can control my pain and stress. I can influence my pain and stress.
> - I can learn to cope better.
> - I feel pain, and it provides me with important information about my body.
> - Pain is not to be avoided, it is to be managed.
> - I view my pain as though it were the rolling surf, a flowing river, or ocean waves coming in and going out. As it moves away from me, I feel relief.
> - I will not fight against the pain, but lie down, relax, and float with it while slowly moving in the direction of relief, tranquility and calm.

In summary, physical and emotional disability need not be devastating or the basis of chronic dysfunctional living. Granted, many people experience events which have had a curtailing influence upon their physical strength and general health. One can approach such situations like these in a passive and defeated manner and essentially submit to the forces that have played a major role in bringing about the state of disability. Alternatively, one can approach such situations from the point of view of recovery and healthy living. Even if one's lifestyle needs to be altered, temporarily or permanently, daily living can be satisfying, meaningful and worth sharing with others. To a large degree, it is a choice. Beyond that, it is determination, direction, and the exercise of a living faith. Go for it!!!

# Chapter Five

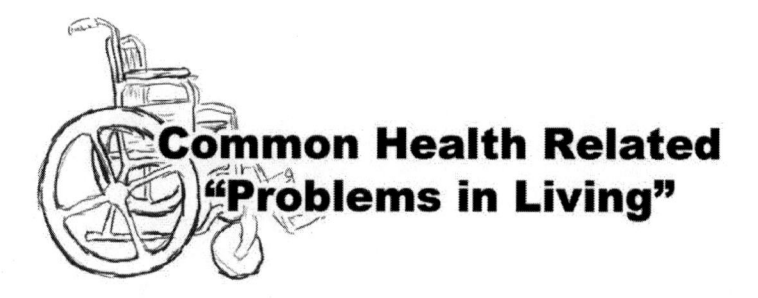

## Common Health Related "Problems in Living"

NO WONDER YOU ARE SICK.
YOU ARE NOT LINKING YOURSELF ENOUGH TO THE
RESOURCES THAT BRING HEALING
*SELWYN HUGHES*

## LIVER LIKES TO BE CARED FOR TOO

Your poor liver never gets any attention; it is a total wallflower located primarily on the right side of the mid body that just quietly takes what you have to dish out. But overlooking this gem is a big mistake because it supports your body in more than 500 ways.

The liver is necessary for survival; there is currently no way to compensate for the absence of liver function long term, although liver dialysis can be used short term. The various functions of the liver are carried out by the liver cells or hepatocytes. Currently, there is no artificial organ or device capable of emulating all the functions of the liver. Some functions can be emulated by liver dialysis, an experimental treatment for liver failure. The liver is thought to be responsible for up to 500 separate functions, usually in combination with other systems and organs.

In Greek mythology, Prometheus was punished by the gods for revealing fire to humans, by being chained to a rock where a vulture would peck out his liver, which would regenerate overnight.

In Plato, and in later physiology, the liver was thought to be the seat of the darkest emotions (specifically wrath, jealousy and greed) which drive men to action. The Talmud refers to the liver as the seat of anger.

The Persian, Urdu, and Hindi languages refer to the liver in figurative speech to indicate courage and strong feelings. "The strength (power) of my liver," is a term of endearment in Urdu. In Persian slang, it is an adjective for any object which is desirable, especially women. In the Zulu language, the word for liver is the same as the word for courage.

*Allan G. Hedberg, Ph.D.*

A clean liver gives you more energy, helps you control your weight and cholesterol levels, and makes you look and feel better. In addition, it regulates sexual arousal, thyroid functioning and the processing of the stress hormones. This organ plays a major role in metabolism and has a number of functions in the body, including glycogen storage, decomposition of red blood cells, plasma protein synthesis, hormone production, and detoxification. Fear not, some of the things that you can do to protect this critical organ are already things you are doing to protect your heart.

To understand how the liver works, it helps to think of it like a filter in a fish tank. Have you ever seen a fish tank that has been neglected? The water is murky and it smells. Everything that you eat, every medication that you take, every breath of toxic air and yes, every sip of alcohol you take has to go through the liver to be processed and eliminated.

Here's what to avoid, and what to add to your diet to keep your liver working at peak performance, according to nutritionist, Theresa Albert.

## Food to Avoid:

1. **Avoid alcohol in excess**. Actually, any amount and any kind of alcohol can damage your liver. Yes, there is evidence that small amounts may protect your heart, but the down side is that it is putting a strain on your liver.
2. **Avoid mixing alcohol and Tylenol**. To make matters worse, if say, you overindulge at a party and take an acetaminophen to try to prevent a headache, you are asking for trouble.
3. **Avoid fatty foods**. All fatty foods have to be processed by the liver, and when this organ gets overwhelmed, it accumulates fat itself (think foie gras). Fatty liver disease can lead to liver inflammation (causing malfunction) and cirrhosis that looks just like the alcoholic sort.
4. **Avoid sugared soft drinks, cakes, pastries, and candy bars**. Dr. Eric Yoshida, Medical Advisor, Canadian Liver

Foundation explains that all of these contain table sugar, which means fructose. "The effect of fructose on the liver cells is similar to alcohol: fat accumulation and oxidation. The current epidemic of non-alcoholic fatty liver disease is because we eat too much table sugar."

5. **Avoid foods that could carry hepatitis.** It might surprise you to hear that raw oysters and undercooked shellfish or pork, pose this serious health risk. Dr. Yoshida said that the pork from Canada or the US is likely to be safe, but pork from other countries like China or Italy has had a history of problems. It may pay to avoid pork if you're unsure of the source.

Preventing liver damage isn't all about what you need to avoid. It also involves a number of foods to ingest and make part of your regular diet.

## Foods to Add:

1. **Add Brazilian nuts, brewer's yeast, kelp, brown rice, garlic, onions and molasses.** These foods are high in selenium, which is required for enzyme activity.
2. **Add eggs, fish, legumes, and seeds.** These foods are high in methionine, which aids in detoxification pathways.
3. **Add broccoli, cauliflower, cabbage and brussels sprouts.** These foods are high in sulfur compounds which aid in detoxification pathways.
4. **Add whole grains, chicken, wheat, bran and nuts.** These foods contain vitamin B5 which speeds up detoxifications of acetaldehyde after alcohol consumption.
5. **Add wheat germ, dried peas and soybeans.** These foods contain vitamin B1 which reduces the toxic effects of alcohol, smoking and lead.

When you take a step back and look at it, these tips make good old common sense and good eating. The difference is now you know what they can do for you in addition to making dinner more pleasurable.

The liver supports almost every organ in the body and is vital for survival. Because of its strategic location and multidimensional functions, the liver is also prone to many diseases.

The most common include: Infections such as Hepatitis A, B, C, E, alcohol damage, fatty liver, cirrhosis, cancer, drug damage (especially acetaminophen, also known as paracetamol, and certain cancer drugs).

Many diseases of the liver are accompanied by the jaundice caused by increased levels of bilirubin in the system. The bilirubin results from the breakup of the hemoglobin of dead red blood cells; normally, the liver removes bilirubin from the blood and excretes it through bile.

There are also many pediatric liver diseases including biliary atresia, alpha-1 antitrypsin deficiency, alagille syndrome, progressive familial intrahepatic cholestasis, and Langerhans cell histiocytosis, to name but a few. Diseases that interfere with liver function will lead to derangement of these processes. However, the liver has a great capacity to regenerate and has a large reserve capacity. In most cases, the liver only produces symptoms after extensive damage.

## Liver Disease Symptoms:

- Pale stools
- Dark urine
- Jaundice
- Swelling
- Excessive fatigue
- Bruising

The liver is the only internal human organ capable of natural regeneration of lost tissue; as little as 25% of a liver can regenerate into a whole liver. It is a "forgiving organ." This is, however, not true for regeneration but rather compensatory growth. The lobes that are removed do not regrow and the growth of the liver is a restoration of function, not original form. This contrasts with true regeneration where both original function and form are restored.

Medical studies about liver regeneration often refer to the Greek Titan Prometheus who was chained to a rock in the Caucasus where, each day, his liver was devoured by an eagle, only to grow back each night. Some think the myth indicates the ancient Greeks knew about the liver's remarkable capacity for self-repair, though this claim has been challenged.

# THE BUDDY SYSTEM FOR LOSING WEIGHT

It is generally well known that Americans have become heavier. Most adults are overweight and many score well into the obesity range. With increased weight, diabetes, high blood pressure, high cholesterol, heart disease, and even premature death can result and place a person at risk.

More recently, we have seen restaurants, schools, and grocery stores place a high value on healthy eating by making conspicuously known the calorie content of various foods and servings. However, schools and restaurants and grocery stores cannot solve the problem alone. Adult and childhood obesity cannot be solved by relying on school policies and restaurant procedures.

For example, it is important to eliminate sugar-flavored milk, cereals, and other food items that have no or little nutritional value, but only contribute significantly to weight gain and a decline in health for both adults and children. We all can promote healthier options by consuming more fresh drinking water in place of flavored milk and other drinks or consume plain, non-fat, 1% milk as well as healthy foods that are high in calcium, especially for older adults and children.

The following array of action steps suggested by the Diet Workshop and others can be taken to help motivate and guide the process of weight loss over the next few months:

*Achieving and Living a Healthy Lifestyle in a World of Stress*

## The Buddy System at Work

- Stand together before a full-length mirror. Take a good look at the chubby twosome, front and sideways, and visualize yourselves as the slim, trim couple you plan to be.
- Enlist a friend to take a picture of the two of you together. Have two prints made. Keep them in prominent places as you go about your respective daily routines.
- Refer to a good weight chart. Study it together and set your individual weight goals.
- Select a good reducing diet. It should be easy to follow, balanced nutritionally, and with enough variety to keep you from getting bored.
- Make a pact that each of one of you will do you best to stick with the diet.
- Plan a week's menu, using the four basic food group, and make up a good marketing list.
- Learn to cook thin together. Use vegetable spray instead of frying in butter or shortening.
- Set your table with smaller plates.
- Observe each other's eating habits and learn to eat slowly, putting down forks between bites.
- Spend some time together preparing low-calorie snacks such as green pepper, carrot and celery sticks and radishes, and keep them refrigerated in ice water wherever you spend your at-home leisure.
- Choose exercises and do them together regularly.
- Set a time to weigh-in together once a week, but no more than once a week.
- Keep individual diaries about your dieting; confess your failures and your success, and suggest to each other ways to improve.
- Remember to compliment each other frequently as you begin to look better and better.
- Reward each other for sticking to the diet, by taking up a new hobby and/or activity you can share.

- Burn calories by an hour of energetic activity. A 120-pound woman can burn up 200-400 calories, 250-500 calories for a 160-pound man.
- Before going out to dinner together, save time to sit down and plan what you'll order—broiled fish, vegetables, salad dressing with diet dressing, fruit cocktail, perhaps a "thin" dessert. Coffee, water, and lots to talk about.
- Treat yourselves to something very special when you've both reached your goals, something (not edible) that your budgets seldom allow, perhaps tickets to a hit show or a sporting event you both enjoy.
- Ask a friend to take another picture of the two of you. Purchase two double frames and place a set of before and after pictures in places where both of you will be reminded frequently of your team triumph.
- Count the number of bites you take per day and keep at 1000 or less. This might be better than counting calories.

Accountability is always a good thing to arrange when trying to change a major problem area in your life. Any addiction is easier to change when accountability partners are in place, according to the Diet Workshop of New York.

# THE BIPOLAR CHALLENGE

SO YOU ARE BIPOLAR!! What a title to give 3% of the adult population. Just what is it? Is it the two extremes of temperament? Is it the two extreme depths of a person's core nature? Is it the extreme of what we all experience when we have moody days? Is it an existential life experience between good and evil? Is it a neurological malady in two parts of the brain? Is it two distinct behavioral patterns learned over time? Unfortunately, we don't fully know. The jury is still out on determining what bipolar is and what causes this behavioral disorder.

Simply stated, a bipolar behavior pattern is the wide range of behaviors and moods a person can exhibit in the course of daily living. We are all capable of being hot one day and cold the next. We are all capable to being vastly excitable and then changing to being grossly serious or somber. Hence, we are all bipolar to a limited degree.

However, those who live at the two extremes of the mood continuum most of their adult life, for whatever reason, are considered to have a Bipolar Disorder. For years we have used a more precise name, which many therapists prefer, Manic Depressive Disorder. To add to the confusing presentation of this disorder, some people live a bipolar life but with less extreme changes over time. Some are mixed and go back and forth between a manic and a depressive mood state.

Allan G. Hedberg, Ph.D.

## The Bipolar Players

Meet Ms/Mr. Manic: These people often have elevated moods, can be extremely irritable or anxious, talk fast and excessively, sleep poorly and exhibit high levels of energy and engage in a variety of impulsive behaviors. They engage in high risk behavior such as gambling and spending sprees and disregard their own health and wellbeing as well as their loved ones, friends and coworkers. For some, energizing hallucinations, paranoia and delusions of grandeur are also present.

Meet Ms/Mr. Depressive: These people live with periodic feelings and thoughts of emptiness, helplessness and sadness. They lack energy and have little interest in anything. Concentration and sustained attention is lacking. Eating, sleeping and most arousal activity are hard to maintain. The "stinking thinking" thoughts of dying and suicide are ever present.

Meet Ms/Mr. Mixed: These people live with a distinct variation in moods over the course of time. Some change daily, weekly or monthly, while others change only once a year or so. They are most venerable to environmental and interpersonal events that may throw them off. They are very difficult to live with and be around for any period of time.

Meet the Doctors: For therapy, psychologists and clinical social workers are the therapists of choice. For the treatment component of medication, psychiatrists and the primary care physician are the medical practitioners of choice. For insurance purposes, a bipolar diagnosis is a parity diagnosis and falls under the medical coverage of the patient's health plan.

## The Bipolar Challenge

The management of the bipolar pattern of behavior is the primary responsibility of the bipolar patient. Helplessness is not an option. Passivity is not acceptable. Also, to do nothing and say, "That's just the way I am" is a total cop out. Such an attitude conveys the message that others must change and accept the bipolar person and personality style. It also says that the bipolar person (patient) is scott-free of any responsibility for his/her behavior. This attitude is self defeating and allows relationships to wither.

On the other hand, bipolar individuals (patients) can live effective and productive lives. They need not live self defeating lives. However, this will largely depend on the actions of the bipolar person and his/her network of support. It is important for the bipolar person to know that to live successfully and to be successful in therapy one must do the following:

- Consistently take the prescribed medication.
- Monitor mood levels daily and take the necessary action steps to stabilize.
- Keep active and maintain a daily routine no matter the mood of the day.
- Set and accomplish specific goals each day.
- Commit to psychotherapy for one year at a time; be faithful to the therapy plan.
- Be around people who are mood stabilizing and encouraging.
- Respect the fact that alcohol and drugs are self destruction.
- Engage in spiritual enrichment and faith building activities
- Engage in self-coaching on how best to behave in any give situation.

Further, bipolar patients must have an active support network. Friends and family make good medicine. Supportive friends and family not only set the expectations but keep the accountability process in place. To live successfully, the support network can aid the patient by assisting in the following manner:

Be a primary source of praise and encouragement for any and all efforts to achieve and moderate moods.

- Hold the patient accountable for agreements, decisions, responsibilities and especially their commitment to therapy.

- Avoid any allowance for excuses for mood changes and irresponsible behavior.
- Go to therapy with the bipolar patient and become part of the healing process.
- Attend a support group for care providers and learn how to manage stress, know more about the bipolar disorder and how to be an agent of change.
- Learn to reinforce and reward "non-bipolar" behavior, such as calmness, rational thinking, productive communication, positiveness and mood moderation.
- Be prepared and have an agreed plan to withhold credit cards and car keys, limit bank account actions, request extra therapy sessions or call in people of authority.
- Be prepared to take constructive and direct action to intervene if the bipolar person suddenly changes.

## The Bipolar Treatment Plan

There are several approaches to the treatment of a bipolar disorder. These include a cognitive-behavioral approach, a neuro-biological approach, and an analytic approach. However, there are a few common themes across all therapies that increase the probability of success. These include but are not limited to the following treatment guidelines:

### TREATMENT GUIDELINES

- Be in psychotherapy while also taking prescribed medication; not just one or the other. In other words, be in therapy, not in the hospital.
- Make changes in therapists and medication until you find a combination of a therapist and a medication that works best for you.
- Admit that a bipolar pattern of life is a significant disorder of thought, mood, and behavioral patterns. All three must be addressed in therapy.

- Admit that a bipolar disorder is a life long challenge that can be managed by following the directions of the doctors with whom there is a working relationship.
- Be sure the therapy program is designed to correct irrational thinking, change the self defeating behavior patterns, teach how to regularly assess and moderate mood and provide reinforcement for every step of improvement.
- Be sure the therapy program teaches Emotional Intelligence and provides guidance in becoming more empathetic, assertive, emotionally self-aware and problem solving, to name a few.
- Avoid alcoholic beverage, cigarettes, street drug use, and only use prescribed medication.
- Expose yourself daily to one to two hours of bright light (sunlight).
- Recognize that the goal is not to cure the bipolar disorder, but to manage symptoms and extreme mood swings to live productively, predictable and evenly.
- Engage in self-coaching; talk to oneself to be calm and moderate at all times.

## The Bipolar Treatment Team Approach

The most recent research finding that makes treatment more likely to succeed is the Team Approach. At no time in history has there been more research evidence indicating that a psychologist serving in the role of therapist and a physician serving in the role of medication management is the most likely "team approach" to succeed.

All across the country we are blessed with a large number of psychotherapists and physicians that have a positive history of working together in a coordinated effort to accomplish the goals of the patient and his or her family. These practitioners are available in the public and in the private sectors of health care in our communities.

Allan G. Hedberg, Ph.D.

## The Bipolar Iceberg

Under the surface of every bipolar patient's emotional state and behavioral pattern is a historical set of strong and influential experiences that carry ongoing feelings of hurt, anger, sadness, loss and abandonment. Such emotion stimulates changes in arousal and produces erratic reaction patterns. If left unresolved, hurts lead to resentment. Unresolved loss leads to depression. Unresolved anger leads to aggression. Unresolved feelings of abandonment lead to a fear of intimacy.

Whatever is under the tip of the iceberg is vitally important. Any and all therapy approaches must discover and understand the unresolved and the unfinished business of one's emotional past. Secondly, the therapist must help create a change of heart and facilitate forgiveness. Without forgiveness, a person can not live in peace or harmony. Without forgiveness, life will be self-defeating and burdened with dissonant or mixed thought and emotions. Without forgiveness, life will tend to be divergent and convex.

## The Bipolar Finale

Keep the patient's eye on the goal. Set the objective and focus on those actions that will help him/her reach their goal. Avoid all actions that will defeat the process of goal attainment. Self-destruction is not an option, self enhancement is the preference. The home, office and community are generally the places where the best healing action takes place; usually not the hospital. The bipolar pattern is manageable and stable living is attainable. To be growing economically, interpersonally, emotionally and spiritually is the primary and focused goal of all parties concerned. Goals, such as moderation, are attainable by behavioral management strategies. Moderation in all things is the key word in the bipolar world.

Previously published in, *The Valley Health Magazine*, August/September, 2007

# MIGRAINE HEADACHES STRIKE AGAIN

A migraine is not your average headache. The pain of a migraine may feel dull, deep, intense or throbbing. That pain often sends migraine sufferers in search of a dark, quiet place to lie down. Untreated, migraines can last from four to 72 hours.

**Prevalence.** An estimated 30 million Americans cope with migraine. About 6%-8% are men and 16%-18% are women. Women outnumber men by 2 or 3 to 1. For China the number is about 1%, and 4.7% for Hong Kong, and 9% in Taiwan.

**Causes.** The cause of migraines isn't fully understood, but both genetic and environmental factors seem to play a role. There are others reasons also. Migraines often run in families.

**Triggers.** Many factors or events may trigger an attack, including high levels of stress; menstruation; use of oral contraceptives; change in weather; going too long without eating; lack of sleep; bright lights, glare, loud noises or strong odors; alcohol; caffeine (too much or withdrawal); and certain foods (aged cheese, cured meats, chocolate, fried foods, and more).

**Medication.** For mild to moderate migraine attacks, over-the-counter medications work well. They are most effective when taken as soon as symptoms begin. Options include aspirin, ibuprofen (Advil, Motrin, others), acetaminophen (Tylenol, others), naproxen sodium (Aleve, others), and combination pain relievers such as Excedrin Migraine. For severe headaches, several prescription medications are options. Consult your physician to select the right one for you.

**Other treatment.** Cognitive behavioral therapy, biofeedback training and relaxation techniques may make migraine medication more effective or reduce the need for it. Getting enough sleep, sticking with a regular schedule, eating regular meals, staying physically active, limiting alcohol and caffeine and managing stress also are important.

Forty minutes of exercise, such as running, was found to be as effective in controlling migraines as was 40 minutes of relaxation exercises and the use of topiramate, a commonly used medicine for migraines. All three procedures helped reduce the frequency of migraines over six months.

Acupuncture is a viable option for those willing to undergo such treatment. No one acupuncture strategy is preferred over another.

**Self control exercise.** Whenever the stress builds up and could result in a headache, engage in a series of self control statements designed to calm the mind and body.

### THE QUIETING RESPONSE EXERCISE

> Whenever you encounter a stressful situation and desire to relax, check your breathing. If it is shallow, indicating tension, say to yourself, "What a silly thing to do to my body." Take a slow and deep breath. Count to five while holding your breath. Exhale slowly to the count of five. Slowly let you breath out and let your body go limp. Imagine your body feeling warm and heavy. Let your jaw droop and relax. Let your neck relax. To help, relax the right hand and arm. Then relax around the neck and down the left arm and hand. Remain still and quiet for a few minutes while increasing the depth of relaxation. Resume your activity

**Prevention.** Preventive treatment can reduce the headache burden by one-third to one-half or more. A doctor can discuss preventive medications that may be helpful, such as blood pressure medications, antidepressants and anti-seizure medications. In addition, injections of Botulinum Toxin type A (Botox) into the scalp muscles can help prevent migraine. Injections need to be repeated every three months. The herbal products feverfew and butterbur may prevent migraine, though the benefits haven't been proved. Supplements of coenzyme Q10 may also be useful for some people. For some, foods that may be helpful include red grapes, soy, cherries, coffee, fish, and turmeric. At the same time, diminish use of processed foods and saturated fats.

Migraines are chronic. Episodes occur anywhere from once or twice a year to once or twice a week. Symptoms can be controlled by working with a primary health care provider and/or a variety of specialists such as, psychologists, chiropractors, bio-feedback therapists, acupuncturist, and others.

# MANAGING GASTROESOPHAGEAL REFLUX DISEASE (GERD)

Reflux means that the stomach acids and juices flow up from the stomach back into the tube that connects the throat and the stomach. This is called the esophagus. This causes heartburn. When you have heartburn at least two times a week, it is called gastroesophageal reflux disease, or GERD. This is a very distressing disorder with much discomfort upon eating.

To minimize and manage the discomfort of the reflux reaction and the associated heartburn, the following behavioral guidelines are recommended. Learn the ones that are most helpful to you.

## Managing GERD Symptoms:

### Eating Patterns

1. Do not eat too much at any given meal.
2. Do not bend forward soon after eating.
3. After eating, wait two to three hours before lying down.
4. Eat smaller meals more often and avoid foods that make you feel distressed.

### Food Selections

5. Avoid coffee, alcohol and excessive amounts of Vitamin C supplements, especially before bedtime.
6. Avoid foods that are high in fats as fat delays stomach emptying.
7. Avoid chocolate and peppermint.

8. Avoid carbonated soft drinks, with or without sugar.
9. Avoid onions, spinach, cabbage, cauliflower, broccoli, brussel sprouts.
10. Avoid drinking milk or eat milk-based products containing calcium and fat within two hours of bedtime.
11. Avoid tomatoes and tomato-based preparations, citrus fruits, and citrus juices.

**Sleep Patterns**

12. Sleep on the left side of your body to reduce night time reflux episodes.
13. Raise the head of your bed six to eight inches by putting blocks under the frame or a foam wedge under the head of the mattress. You may also use extra pillows.

**Lifestyle Factors**

14. Lose weight.
15. Quit smoking or using tobacco.
16. Wear loose-fitting clothing around your waist and mid-section to put less pressure on the stomach.
17. Use chewing gum or hard candies to increase the amount of saliva your mouth produces. Saliva washes stomach juices out of the esophagus into the stomach and can control stomach acid.
18. Use over-the-counter anti-acid medication. If this does not work sufficiently, consult your physician for a prescriptive medication.

Be sure you are under the care of a physician for this disorder and follow any medical advice given you. While all these efforts may not lead to a cure, some relief is better than living with the basic problem of GERD being unaddressed.

# MANAGING CHRONIC PAIN

## Start with Helping Yourself

Even when pain lingers on and on, there are ways of making yourself feel better. Printed below is a treatment program that has worked for many people with pain problems similar to yours. Your doctor can help you tailor the plan to your specific needs. Keep this sheet handy as a reminder of the general principles.

The goals of this program are to:

1. Reduce the amount of medication you are taking or eliminate it altogether.
2. Reduce your pain.
3. Increase your activity level.
4. Return you to work/school.

To meet these program goals, follow these four guidelines:

1. **Realize that although others can try to help, only you can make yourself feel better**. Your doctor and family can give advice and support, but you have to assume responsibility for relieving your pain and taking an active role in the management of your pain related problem.
2. **Gradually decrease the amount of medication you take.** Pain relievers rarely help lingering pain. After you have taken a pain medication for a long time, your body develops tolerance, so the drug no longer provides relief. It may make you feel better, but this is because your body has become dependent on the medication. Due to this dependence, your doctor will not stop the medication abruptly. He will slowly

*Achieving and Living a Healthy Lifestyle in a World of Stress*

     reduce the amount of medication you take, giving your body a chance to get used to being without the medication.
3. **Focus on your activities rather than your pain**. Try to stop thinking and talking about how much you hurt. Such talk will only make you feel worse. Becoming more active and thinking and talking about what you're doing will help you take your mind off your pain. Talking about activities encourages more activity.
4. **Gradually increase your level of activity.** Unless your doctor has a reason to advise against it, activity is not harmful. Acute pain, such as that from an ankle sprain, is a warning sign that rest is needed. However, when pain has continued for several months, the presence of pain does not necessarily mean something bad will happen if you move.

Your doctor will help you set up a program of gradually increasing activity, starting with what you are able to do comfortably right now. Plan to do a certain amount each day. In other words, set a quota. Increase that quota slightly over the next few days. An increase by 10% is the rule of thumb for increasing your progress. Avoid the trap of starting or stopping an activity according to how you feel. You will find it helpful to keep a record of how much you do each day in an "activity diary."

For many people, walking, biking and swimming are a few of the best activities, regardless of where the pain is located. Your doctor will also recommend exercises that strengthen the muscles in the areas of your body where you have pain.

This program may sound simple—it offers no miracle drugs, no new operations—but it has helped many people. Even if your pain doesn't go away completely, just think about all you're able to do that you thought you couldn't do! Hopefully, you will be able to do more in the days ahead. Follow the program.

*Allan G. Hedberg, Ph.D.*

## Allowing Others to Help

With medical assistance, your, spouse, family member, relative, or friend, can be of great help with managing your pain if you allow them to follow the program outlined below, developed by specialists in the management of pain and has worked for many people with similar problems. The goals are to reduce pain, cut down the amount of medication being taken, and increase the level of physical activity. In order to succeed, your help will be required. You may not like what the program calls for and how others are to interact with you. However, follow the program and let the benefits come in time.

Below are the instructions for anyone desiring to help a person with chronic pain:

1. **Do not talk about pain.** When talking about the chronic pain, the pain will feel more intense and will lead to the perception that things are getting worse. Try these suggestions:
    - When he/she starts talking about his/her pain, let him/her finish the statement, but try to divert his/her attention by introducing a new subject when he pauses for breath.
    - When he/she talks about his/her pain, break eye contact.
    - Avoid asking about the pain. Instead, focus on the activities in which he/she have been engaged. For instance, when you return from work or shopping, don't ask how he/she feels, but ask what he/she did while you were gone.
2. **Help increase their level of activity. Activity is not harmful even if it hurts.** Only acute pain, such as that due to a sprain or strain, requires rest. After pain has continued for several months, the presence of pain upon movement usually means that part of the body is stiff and weak from disuse. As the muscles get back into shape and use, the pain will most likely diminish.

    The doctor or physical therapist will help set an exercise goal. The amount of activity should increase each day. An increase of 10% is a good rule to follow. After the activity

level goes up, the pain level will probably go down. But many people who follow this program resume an active life even if the pain persists. As a "cheerleader" or support person, your role is to:
- Give encouragement by praising increases in activity and urging him/her on when he/she seems to be faltering.
- Plan interesting activities both in and out of the home.
- Avoid "rewarding" him/her by attending to, responding to, or sympathizing with the complaints of pain.

3. **Praise all improvements in "pain-managing" behavior.** Efforts to increase activity, lower drug use, talking about non-pain oriented topics, and not reflecting on how life is better are all worthy of praise. Any and all non-pain, non-disability, and non-despair topics of discussion should be immediately affirmed and praised. It is vital that the person with chronic pain be strongly encouraged to think and talk about other topics than pain. Over time, if pain topics are not allowed or given interest, the person will soon begin to talk on other topics and think more positively. As a "cheerleader" or support person your role is to:
- Listen for positive and non-pain talk and respond to it favorably
- Ask questions and encourage talk about daily activities, projects engaged in, and hobbies/interests pursued.
- Set an example by talking more positively yourself and having a positive image.
- Be willing to do some activity during your visit or intentionally direct your efforts to be devoted towards increased behavioral activities of interest to the chronic pain patient. Be prepared to be active, not just sit and talk.

Chronic pain is tough to live with and tough to endure as a by-stander, family member or otherwise. However, it only gets worse with inactivity, depression, isolation, complaining, and lack of stimulation. As a "cheerleader" support person you are able to reverse the trend and get more activity, energy, interest and hope. It is not easy, to be sure. It takes intentional effort and time. Do not give up. Be creative. Consult others who are in a similar situation. Join a support group or interest group for your own good and for ideas to try. Be careful not to burnout as a care provider. Take care of yourself and provide care as you are able for the loved one in your life who is living with chronic pain.

## Common Errors Made by Pain Patients

Below are several common mistakes in the thinking of pain patients regarding their management of pain and the use of medication.

1. **Pain medication is not to block all pain at all times.** The use of medication in pain management is to give about 50-60% relief and all reasonable activity. Accepting a limited amount of pain and coping with it is part of the self-management of pain.
2. **Pain medication is not to be taken whenever pain is felt and whenever a flare-up occurs.** Mediation is best used on a time schedule, not whenever you feel like it. Further, over and frequent use will only use up the supply of pills and leave none for later when the may be needed.
3. **Pain is not all physical.** Pain is the combination of a physical condition and a person's perception of a state of discomfort. It is also related to a person's belief that pain is bad and a sign that something very serious is wrong in the body and will only get worse.
4. **Pain medication needs to be refilled on schedule and not the last minute.** If one waits too long for a refill, it might not be possible to arrange for the refill and a period of time of no medication may have to be endured.
5. **Pain medication is not the only management tool.** Pain is also handled by taking breaks every 30 minutes, learning to engage in relaxation procedures, focusing on non-pain thoughts and activities, walking, joining a pain management support group, visualizing relaxing scenes and images, and pacing your activities over the day, to name a few.

Remember, it is the management of chronic pain, not the elimination of it. It takes time and consistent effort to achieve a good level of control. Keep yourself calm and relaxed. Gradually build your strength back. Believe in yourself once again.

# INSOMNIA: What is it and what can we do about it?

There is little question that insomnia is real. It is a significant problem for 37 million Americans over 55 years of age who do not get enough of deep restorative sleep to function well. Studies demonstrate that 13 percent of the male population and 26 percent of the female population complain of insomnia. Insomnia is no respecter of person or age. It is found among all ethnic groups. With increasing age, our need for sleep remains about the same but the quality of sleep slowly deteriorates. Brain wave pattern become more irregular with increasing age and sleep also become irregular. Insomnia is generally understood to be a significant sleep disorder if it occurs four or more times per week.

Sleep disorder researchers agree on six factors that contribute to insomnia. They are:

1. Underlying biological factors.
2. Underlying psychological factors.
3. Drug and alcohol use.
4. Disturbing environmental factors
5. Negative sleep related learning experiences.
6. Pre-sleep and sleep habits.

**What You Do About It:**

There have been many strategies proposed for the treatment of insomnia. For many people, the focus is placed on biological factors. For them medication therapies are thought to be the be all and end all of this problem. Unfortunately, medications to aid sleep are not the answer for most people. Sleep medication can interact with other medications and create other problems. They can hide or cover up other medical conditions needing medical attention. They can impair motor and cognitive functioning if used over an extended period of time.

For others, insomnia is considered to be a result of learned behavior. For such individuals, there is a need to unlearn certain patterns of behavior associated with insomnia and learn new behavioral patterns associated with healthy sleep habits.

Others approach insomnia with a strong belief in the power of "pre-sleep" and sleep habits. Some specific home remedies or prohibitions are the answer for them. For example, coffee is not to be consumed after 6:00 p.m. Certain bedtime rituals must be followed obsessively.

There are as many answers for insomnia as there are people that ask. We all think we know the answer. However, each sleeper must find his/her own answer and then stick with it. Research has indicated that there are some generally accepted strategies that help many people.

Whatever approach is adopted, it is important to start out with the selection of a mattress that fits the weight and frame of your body and your sleep style preference. Many new types of mattresses have been developed in recent years. Find one that works best for you. Bed linens are also a strong consideration. For some, sleep is facilitated by the material of the sheets utilized. If a pad is utilized, it is important that the pad be stabilized and held in a smooth and comfortable position.

**Helpful Hints for Easing into Sleep:**

1. If you do not fall asleep within 20 minutes, get out of bed and engage in some relaxing activity for 20 minutes. Return to bed and proceed through your pre-sleeping routine.

However, if you are not sleeping within 20 minutes, get out of bed again and repeat the relaxing activity. After 20 minutes return back to bed and engage in your pre-sleeping routine. Repeat this procedure throughout the night until you fall asleep. Continue this routine for at least 30 days.
2. Exercise in the mornings or afternoons but not immediately before bedtime. However, a light evening stroll for relaxation purposes could be helpful.
3. Nap during the day, but restrict it to one hour and at the same time each day, preferably between noon and 4:00 p.m., as this is the body's natural down time.
4. Do not consume caffeine beverages such as coffee, chocolate, mocha, sodas and tea after 6:00 p.m. Evening alcohol consumption and smoking is not recommended.
5. Use sleeping pills under a physician's directions and usually not for more than a month or two to break the cycle of insomnia.
6. Do not eat a large meal within an hour or two of bedtime. A light evening meal is recommended.
7. Develop a pre-sleeping routine such as proceeding through a series of relaxation exercises, listening to music, writing in a daily journal or taking a shower or bath. The use of the radio as part of pre-sleep routine may be helpful to distract interfering thoughts.
8. A bed is for sleeping so don't use it as a place for eating, watching television, reading or carrying out an argument.
9. Room temperature and air quality may be important for sleep. Determine what is the best temperature for you and maintain that temperature in the bedroom all night.
10. Sleep the same hours each night of the week. Remember that while 7 or 8 hours of sleep is desirable, the body can function on 6 hours of sleep.
11. Some herbal teas have been found to be soothing. Some may have sedative qualities.
12. If you suspect sleep apnea due to your heavy snoring, gasping for air while sleeping, and frequent brief sleep interruptions, consider consulting a medical sleep clinic.

13. If you are a person who worries and becomes stressed regarding problems in living, do not work on worrisome or stressful projects within an hour of bedtime.
14. Use imagery to your advantage. Select an image that will help you fall asleep. Images commonly used are, a burning candle, a favorite vacation scene, clouds, a pleasant fantasy, waterfalls, floating on or sinking into a mattress.
15. Use a muscle relaxation procedure in which five or six muscle groups are sequentially tensed and held tense for 5 seconds and then relaxed. Do this over a 10 to 15 minute period of time starting with the feet and legs and proceeding to the head.
16. Should you choose to have a late night snack, it would be best to select foods that are rich in L-tryptophane, an amino acid that may contribute to improve sleep patterns. A sample of night time snack food products would be milk, eggs, cottage cheese, soy beans, tuna, and turkey.
17. Engage in a mental activity that exercises both sides of the brain simultaneously. The left side of the brain processes a lineal sequence of information such as saying the alphabet, counting numbers or lining up objects from simple to complex or from small to large. The right side of the brain processes the visual representation of an activity and creates the visual image of the activity, such as swimming or dancing. Hence, both parts of the brain are active simultaneously and may serve to distract the brain from thoughts that would compete with sleep. Hence, count backwards or say the alphabet backwards while visualizing numbers or letters being written on a large blackboard in your mind.

## The Role of a Mid-Day Nap

Some people find a mid-day nap helpful while others do not. It is important if you have insomnia to go to bed and wake up at the same time each night. It is also important if you do take a nap that you do so at the same time each day such as mid afternoon, but only nap for one hour. This is called a "power nap." Do not sleep for lengthy periods of time. Be sure to program your day so that you will stay awake throughout the day other than the time taken for the power nap of one hour. Be sure to have a regular bedtime.

## Professional Consultation

By all means, professional consultation and intervention would be helpful to overcome a genuine sleep disorder, such as insomnia. As indicated above, there are many reasons for insomnia. There are also many alternative professional treatment approaches that can be utilized besides the informal approaches as noted above.

A person with insomnia may benefit from different professional consultations and treatment approaches, such as, biofeedback training, acupuncture, chiropractic services, massage and a referral to a medical sleep clinic. Whatever approach is utilized, it is important to pursue it for at least a few months before considering a different alternative.

## Factors Affecting Sleep

Sleep patterns are enhanced by the general happiness level of an individual or group of people. In other words, the better the physical, mental and emotional health of an individual, the better the quality of sleep. Times of unrest such as unemployment or worrisome situations interfere with quality sleep.

## Learning More about Sleep

The following internet websites would be good sources to consult:

1. **www.talkaboutsleep.com** After accessing the site, click on Sleep Basics.
2. **www.sleepfoundation.org**

# ATTENTION-DEFICIT DISORDERS AND HYPERACTIVITY

An attention disorder with or without hyperactivity (ADHD) can be diagnosed in young children as young as 4 years of age. It is generally believed that the sooner a treatment plan can be initiated, the more likely the child will benefit and avoid pitfalls of academic failure and social misbehavior. Usually treatment commences by age 6. It is now believed that children as young of 4 would benefit significantly from a systematic treatment approach if their behavior is outside the bounds of typical 4-year-olds, according to the American Academy of Pediatrics. ADHD is diagnosed when children are overactive, impulsive, distractible, prone to accidents, and do not play well with other children. They are known for their inability to focus or pay attention. Behavior patterns are not consistent from day-to-day.

The brains of ADHD children mature normally, but may take up to three years longer to fully develop. The caudate nucleus and the frontal area of the brain's cortex control the functions of attention, reasoning, planning, and memory. Problems in learning relate to this area of the brain especially. Once the full development takes place, the ADHD fades and learning takes place with greater ease, for most of the children. Some will continue to live with the attention and concentration problems for years to come.

ADHD children need a systematic treatment approach which includes medication and the teaching of behavioral management techniques to both parents and the child. The behavior management techniques to be utilized involve the following:

1. A reward system for acceptable behavior.

2. Stress management procedures to teach emotional control and management.
3. Relaxation training to teach muscle relaxation and calmness.
4. Visual focusing training to teach attention and concentration.
5. Teach children to walk slowly, talk slowly, eat slowly, and engage in other daily behaviors slowly, as if they were a turtle.
6. Learn to disregard extraneous noises, movements, and sights, so the child can learn to disregard distractions and focus one's attention.
7. Set in place a discipline plan to stop and /or change inappropriate behavior.

Medication is generally needed by ADHD children, at least on a trial basis for three to four months. It is common to start with one medication and change to another, or start at one dosage level and increase it to the next highest dosage level. For young children, Ritalin is most commonly used for moderate and severe ADHD children. Concerta is generally the second choice with young children and the primary choice with older children, 6 to 12 years of age. Some children require medication for at least a year and others until they reach the mid-adolescent years. Some need medication beyond the teen years and into their young adult years.

Drugs such as Ritalin, Concerta and other such medications fall within the stimulant category of medication and appear to boost and balance the brain chemicals called neurotransmitters. Not only do such medications address symptoms of inattention and hyperactivity, but also facilitates improved cognitive processing of information. There are other medications available to consider and this should be well discussed with the psychologist and the physician.

To be properly diagnosed, a child is generally monitored over a three to six-month period of time, and observed in at least two different environments such as the home and classroom, preschool or day care center. As part of the evaluation of a child, parents need to be interviewed along with the child's teacher or day care provider.

There are questionnaires and behavioral assessment techniques that can be utilized as part of the evaluation process.

Research seems to indicate that children who go untreated are at risk for academic problems, social problems, and significant interpersonal difficulties. This possibility of problems is not only true during their childhood years but also well into their adolescent and young adult years.

Children with inattention and hyperactivity are generally evaluated and treated by the child's pediatrician, clinical psychologist, and teacher along with the parents all working together as a team. Any of these professionals would be a good starting point for parents that have a child suspected of inattention and hyperactivity.

# HEARING LOSS CONTRIBUTES TO DEPRESSION AND DEMENTIA

The loss of hearing is not a simple matter as it seems. Over the years, those that have experienced hearing loss have had to learn to live with it, compensate for it, accommodate to it, or improve their hearing through the use of various hearing aid devices. Those who experience deafness or near-deafness must deal with this problem in a more exaggerated manner. Recent research indicates that the person undergoing a loss of hearing must not only deal with the frustrations of inadequate hearing for the social occasion, but must also deal with the depression and the cognitive loss that results from suppressed hearing and deafness. A reliance on our hearing for social interaction and learning is basic to our moods and the cognitive processing of information. Without adequate hearing, we withdraw and isolate, and reduce our social interactions. This all suppresses feelings of happiness, pleasure, and enjoyment. When hearing is reduced, we experience less stimulation to the brain resulting in a loss of brain functions and the processing of information necessary for new learning, memory, and alert interaction with the environment. Dementia is more likely to develop.

Hearing loss is the experience of 30% of the population 65 years of age and older, and 75% of those 85 years of age and older. Hence, there is a direct correlation between hearing loss and age, and a slow progression of hearing loss with age.

In a recent research study conducted at the Mt. Sinai Alzheimer's Disease Research Center and published in the February, 2011 issue of *Archives of Neurology*, it was found among those over 60 years of age that 36% experienced an increased dementia risk directly related to hearing loss. The greater the hearing loss, the greater the chance of being diagnosed with dementia. For every additional loss of ten decibels of hearing capacity, dementia appeared to increase by 20%.

How can this be? We hear as a result of tiny hair cells located in the inner ear that transforms environmental sound waves into nerve impulses. The brain then interprets the pattern of impulses as speech, the sound of a whistle, a dog barking, or the whisper of the wind. These patterns are learned as a result of a complex series of associations that have been set up over the years between an environmental sound and a particular brain pattern of impulses.

As we grow older, the tiny cells in the auditory portion of the brain die off or are damaged. This means that the structure of the ear become less responsive to sound waves resulting in the loss of hearing, especially in certain ranges. This is called Age-Related Hearing Impairment (ARHI).

It is possible that the damage to nerve cells relates to direct exposure to loud sounds or to the non-use or lack of stimulation over time. It is also possible that the brain reallocates resources to help with hearing at the expense of cognition. They also may be indirectly related to the cardiovascular health of an individual with a combination of such problems. Cardiovascular ill health and loss of brain cell usage, leads directly to dementia.

As noted above, the loss of hearing also contributes to depression. Social isolation and the lack of social engagement and stimulation allows the brain to malfunction, creating advanced stages of dementia. The lack of social stimulation contributes directly to the loss of stimulation and enrichment of the brain itself, placing the brain at risk for dementia. People become discouraged and depressed as they withdraw and isolate, as well as have increased difficulty hearing and processing information. It is a vicious cycle of neurological, social and cognitive dysfunction. Certainly, one affects the other.

*Allan G. Hedberg, Ph.D.*

## Dealing with Hearing Loss

1. Schedule a hearing evaluation by an audiologist.
2. Arrange to obtain hearing aids for both ears. The more that you are socially active, the more sophisticated hearing aid is required.
3. Change your phone system so that an enhanced hearing volume option is available for your use.
4. Let others know that you have hearing aids in the same way that you wear glasses, or paint your fingernails.
5. Socialize with others whenever there is opportunity.
6. Stay physically active to challenge your brain.

The mere improvement of hearing through the use of hearing aids and other procedures will not cure or reverse one's state of dementia. However, the advancement of dementia can be slowed through the use of hearing aids and other procedures.

In summary, we are rapidly coming to the point where dementia affects over a hundred million people. While the state of dementia is not reversible, it can be delayed by a year or more by carrying out certain procedures for brain stimulation, enrichment, and complexity of interaction. Dementia is easier to prevent than to reverse. It is easier to slow its process rather than reverse it. Previous research seems to indicate that dementia is facilitated by social isolation, a sedentary lifestyle, and certain health problems such as cardiovascular difficulties, diabetes, hypertension, and other types of health problems. We now come to a point in our research where we note that hearing loss may well be a contributor to the development of dementia. Thankfully, hearing loss can be addressed and altered, particularly if it is caught early following onset.

# DEPRESSION PLACES WOMEN AT RISK FOR A STROKE

A stroke is one of the most devastating neurological events that can happen to a person. Usually a stroke is perpetrated by a blood vessel in the brain bursting, causing diffuse bleeding, manifest by a significant weakness or total dysfunction of one side of the body or the other, among other physical features. Depressed women may face an increased risk of stroke, according to a recent article by Dr. Kathryn Rexrode, published in *Stroke, A Journal of the American Heart Association.*

Dr. Rexrode followed over 80,000 women, ages 54 to 79, over six years to determine the effects of depression on their potential to have a stroke. Women who used antidepressant medication, such as selective serotonin reuptake inhibitors (SSRIs), such as Prozac, Zoloft and Celexa, were compared to those women who were depressed but did not use such medication. Those participating in the study were predominantly white registered nurses. All of them were without a prior history of stroke. All were assessed over six years on multiple occasions with a Mental Health Index. Depression was defined as those currently reporting or having a history of depression symptoms.

The reported prevalence of depression among these women at baseline was 22%. Over the six years, the researchers found that a history of depression was associated with a 29% increased risk of total stroke, even after considering other stroke risk factors. Women who used antidepressant medication, particularly the SSRI medication, had a 39% increased risk of stroke.

Compared to women without a history of depression, depressed women were more likely to be single, smokers, and less physically

*Allan G. Hedberg, Ph.D.*

active. Further, they were also slightly younger, had a higher Body Mass Index, and more co-existing health conditions such as high blood pressure, heart disease and diabetes. It was further found that those with depression found that their depression interfered with their ability to control certain medical problems such as diabetes, hypertension, and other medical problems. For example, they found it difficult to exercise. They found that mood was often an interference to live a routine and healthy lifestyle. All these factors contributed to increased risk for stroke.

Dr. Rexrode was quick to state that antidepressant medication use may be an indicator of depression severity but she did not think that the medication itself was a primary cause of the risk. The research study did not suggest that people should stop their antidepressant medication or other medications to reduce their risk of stroke.

The occurrence of a stroke may be linked to other factors such as inflammation or an underlying vascular disease in the brain. It may also be related to the intake of an antioxidant diet, such as high grains, fruits and veggies. Based on a Swedish study, The American Heart Association encourages diets high in antioxidants as a way to lower risk of stroke, even among women with a history of cardiovascular disease.

Regardless of the mechanism by which a stroke occurs, recognizing that depressed individuals may be at a higher risk of stroke may help physicians focus on treating the depression and treating stroke risk factors such as hypertension, diabetes, and elevated cholesterol. These research findings may encourage physicians to prompt their patients to address adverse lifestyle behaviors such as smoking and the lack of exercise. A referral to a mental health professional may be the better part of valor. Preventative strategies needs to be strongly advocated, particularly among depressed women and those that have depression along with signs and symptoms of higher risk of stroke. It is essential that anyone with a history of depression not go untreated, preferably by both medication and personal counseling.

# CORONARY HEART DISEASE AND LIFESTYLE

In the United States, it is estimated that over 4,600,00 people are victims of heart disease, and over 560,000 people die annually from various forms of coronary heart disease. Coronary artery disease is the most common type of heart disease and is one of the leading causes of death. Coronary artery disease is the result of fatty deposits which block the arteries that carry oxygenated blood and nutrients to the heart muscle as well as elsewhere throughout the body. If the condition is severe and/or continues over time, there can be damage to the heart and a heart attack will likely occur with little notice.

**Risk Factors:**

A. Major risk factors that cannot be changed.

1. Hereditary—There is a familiar tendency toward heart disease or Arteriosclerosis.
2. Sex—Men are at greater risk than women of having a heart attack.
3. Race—There is a 45% greater chance among Blacks than Whites having high blood pressure.
4. Age—More than one in five heart attacks occur before age 65.

B. Major risk factors that can be changed.

1. Cigarette Smoking—Smokers have twice the risk of heart attacks than non-smokers and it is the most prevalent risk factor in sudden cardiac death. The risk of heart disease

is rapidly reduced when smoking is terminated, regardless how long one has smoked.
2. High Blood Pressure—It is the "silent killer" which adds to the heart's workload, thereby enlarging and weakening the heart over a long period of time.
3. Blood Cholesterol Levels—Too much cholesterol in the blood can cause fat build-up on the walls of the arteries, narrowing and eventually closing off the flow of blood eventually leading to a heart attack or stroke.
4. Diabetes—Diabetes can escape detection for years, but can sharply increase a person's risk of heart attack.

C. Contributing Factors

1. Obesity—It places a heavy burden on your heart, influences muscular strength, blood pressure, blood cholesterol and precipitating diabetes.
2. Lack of Exercise—This contributes to poor stamina, endurance, and weakens heart functioning.
3. Stress—Poorly managed excessive and chronic stress over a long period of time may create heart related problems.

## Lifestyle Challenges:

A. Quit smoking for good.
B. Have your blood pressure checked annually after age 40, and more often if a problem develops.
C. Exercise regularly—A half hour of fairly strenuous exercise daily will strengthen your heart. Your body will function more efficiently and you can manage physical and emotional stress with regular exercise and other measures more effectively.
D. Diet and lose those extra pounds.—Reduce foods high in saturated fats, cholesterol, salty foods and snacks.
E. Modify your "Type A" behavior—. Reduce your behavioral emphasis on time urgency, feelings of hostility, tension and a competitive spirit. (See below)

F. Daily practice stress reduction—Reduce stress from your environment by taking time to relax. If you have not learned to relax, the use of relaxation training tapes and CDs, and biofeedback training can be helpful.
G. Consider personal counseling—Research has shown that 5-10 sessions significantly reduces patterns of ill-health and its associated risks.

If you have identified some medical risk factor, consult a physician and a psychologist to make the necessary changes in your lifestyle.

In conclusion, the Serenity Prayer says it most aptly. It reads as follows, *"May God grant me the serenity to accept the things I cannot change; the courage to change the things I can; and wisdom to know the difference."*

## ARE YOU A TYPE "A" PERSON?

1. Do you accent certain words when speaking—even in casual conversation?
2. Do you move, talk, eat rapidly?
3. Do you show impatience with others' slowness—even interrupt their conversation with you, "yes, yes," etc.?
4. Do you engage in polyphasic thinking and action? (That is, two things at once).
5. Do you pretend to pay attention, yet let your mind wander to your own thoughts?
6. Do you feel guilty if you are not working?
7. Do you not see the beauty around you because you are too busy?
8. Are you busy getting things worth having, as opposed to becoming a being of worth?
9. Do you have a chronic sense of urgency for time?
10. Does another type "A" arouse your hostility?
11. Do you clench you fists and bang, when you are upset?
12. Do you do things faster than others?
13. Do you measure worth by numbers?

# Chapter Six

## Aging as a Class Act in Finishing Well

YOUTH IS MADE RICH BY THE DREAMS OF THE FUTURE;
AGE IS MADE POOR BY ITS REGRETS FOR THE PAST
*ROCHEPEDRE*

# WHAT IS THIS ABOUT MEN DYING BEFORE WOMEN?

On the block on which my family lives, there are twenty-one homes. We moved to our present home in 1974. The neighborhood consisted of all young parents raising their families at the time. Now, we are all in our senior years enjoying the experience of rearing grandchildren.

Over the years, our neighborhood experienced the death of eleven men and two women. All but one died as a result of aging and the usual high frequency chronic illnesses of cancer and heart disease. One died in an industrial accident. Why the discrepancy? Why do men die earlier than women? Is it due to where they live or it is genetic and/or cultural factors?

Statistics indicate that that those that live to 100 years, women outnumber men about eight to one. Overall, women over the age of 65 will outlive men by three years. The oldest person of modern times was Jeanne Calment, of Paris, who lived to age 122 years. In considering these facts, we must consider the effects of estrogen, menstruation-related toxic elimination, the X chromosome, job related stress, disease survival, levels of social behavior, and the tendency to eat healthier diets. All these factors may all play a role in why women live longer than men.

Consider some of the facts related to health and longevity. Men are much less likely than women to look after their health and visit physicians. They are 25% less likely to have visited a physician in the last year, and are about 40% more likely to have skipped cholesterol screening and similar health care maintenance wellness procedures according to the U.S. Agency for Health Care Research

*Allan G. Hedberg, Ph.D.*

and Quality. Men go to doctors and get diagnostic work-ups because of the nagging of their wife and children. Further, there are many medical clinics and specialists for women, but not for men.

As men tend to be in poorer health, they are one and a half times more likely to die from heart disease, cancer, respiratory diseases, and similar disorders, according to the U.S. Centers for Disease Control and Prevention. They die on the average five years earlier than women. On the other hand, men are less likely to experience Alzheimer's disease, are generally healthier, and have better cognitive functioning.

There may be a genetic component. Some variation of the Y chromosome may make men more prone to heart disease, it is believed.

A man's life span may be related to socialization factors within the culture. Men tend not to socialize and benefit from social interaction and support as do women. Research has shown an array of traits that may contribute to men's early demise. For example, men tend to suppress emotional expressions, be more aggressive, and take greater risks which places their life and health in jeopardy.

Can men learn to live a healthier lifestyle and live longer? There are men who are known for certain masculine traits that make them more prone to visit their physicians and avoid risky behaviors. These favorable masculine traits are self-reliant, responsibility, emotional maturity, and being even-keeled. These are traits worthy of development in any man, of any race, and of any faith orientation.

## Men Need to Rethink Their Self Image

What will it take for men to learn to care for themselves and maintain a healthy lifestyle? Consider the following factors:

1. While it is generally considered to be wimpy and unmasculine for men to be concerned about their health, in fact, men

really are concerned about their health. It is acceptable for men to be health conscious and take steps to achieve and maintain a healthy lifestyle. Men need to learn to be more human and vulnerable.

2. Research supports the notion that men are less knowledgeable about health and, therefore, put themselves at risk and do not take adequate care of themselves. Health education is a key activity for men to engage in if they are going to protect and advance their health. Health education includes the use of helmets, seat belts, driving patterns, adrenaline seeking behavior, age appropriate risk taking, and aggressive play. These are all areas that would benefit a man if he were to engage in a positive and systematic health education program.

3. It is not uncommon for men to think of themselves as being immune to disease, injury, and common illness. This type of irrational thinking needs to drastically change so men will come to accept their humanness and vulnerability to germs, diseases, and risk-related accidents. They need to learn to take precautions accordingly. They need to believe that the worse could happen to them as well.

4. Men tend to have fewer friends and a much smaller social support network than women. Social support has always been a contributing factor to positive health. All men, but especially singles, need to engage in social network support building, such as forming a golfing foursome, joining a service club in the community, joining in on an early morning coffee clutch at the local restaurant, and attending a church with services geared to their age group. Men need to work more intentionally at building a social network of support.

5. It is not uncommon for men to take care of their car better than they take care of their own bodies. Men need to accept the fact that as cars need tune-ups so does their body, especially their brain and their heart. Men need to plan for and engage in body tune-ups.

6. Men like to be in charge. Men tend to be achievement oriented, competitive. The key factor is for men to learn how to take control of their life and behavior patterns for

the purpose of beating disease, illness, and various forms of physical impairments. Men not only need to achieve academically and vocationally but also live healthfully. By taking control of their health status, men can beat a disease or illness that otherwise would take root.

In summary, men might respond better to health messages and participate more fully and willingly in health care screening, diagnostic procedures and treatment if their masculinity is not perceived to be violated.

One of the key factors of masculinity is the challenge of asking for help. Asking for help is a difficult thing for any man to do. Those that are able to ask, enter into the health keeping process more openly and sooner. The risk for being impaired or dying is lessened accordingly. Hence, health care seeking is an act of self-reliance. Taking charge of one's health is what it really means to be a real man. And real men engage in and become a partner in their own care along with their family and the health care community. Men have decision making power about their health as they do about other areas in their life. They just need to learn to exercise it

# THE LONG JOURNEY OF AGING

The aging process involves a long and arduous journey on a pathway with many pot holes and unknowns. The journey takes some through the valley of death. For others, life is lived in the shadows of loneliness. The depths of depression and anxiety are an ever present experience for many. Thankfully, for others, the journey is relatively positive with many scenic points of interest, stimulation, encouragement, and support. The following guidelines may be helpful in relating to and helping an aging family member in his/her journey through his/her final decades of life.

1. **Focus efforts on staying connected.** It is important that an aging individual remain connected with the people, things, places and memories of their past. These are all subjects for good discussion. Success in keeping the individual involved in some aspects of his/her historical experience can be a source of pleasure and encouragement.
2. **Listen to their stories of grief and loss** Do not feel sorry for what has happened in their past. It is important that the aging person have opportunity to share their grief and tell of their loss experiences. Listen and express compassion. Also, empathy and support would be appreciated.
3. **Know that there is an open door for asking questions.** Older people love to tell about themselves and their experiences in the past. Feel free to ask specific questions. Inquire about their current situation or if there is a present need that should be addressed. Offer help if you are able to do so. If not, engage someone who can be of assistance.
4. **Ask about their deceased spouse, children, family members and friends**. Be sensitive to their feelings as they respond to your inquiry. Do not prolong the discussion

unless the individual takes the lead and carries on the conversation.

5. **Engage in a meaningful activity together to increase socialization.** It is acceptable to invite or nudge a person into an activity that helps them connect with others. In addition, the feelings of loneliness should decrease as the opportunity for new friendships to develop. Resistance may occur but continue to pursue the activity. Over time, they will eventually accept your invitation. He or she may eventually look forward to the activity when you visit.

6. **Accept where they are at this point of life**. Some may have had a lifetime of dysfunctional relationships, pain, hurt, and trauma. Older folk tend to be "set in their ways." Accept them for who they are and for how they handle events, situations and people. Change does not come easily for them.

7. **Tell the older person that you have been thinking about them**. We all love to hear that we are in the thoughts of people who love us and are part of our world. It is even better to go beyond and specify what thoughts had been brought to your attention and what those thoughts mean to you.

8. **Do something special together at any time, but especially on special occasions.** Consider going for a walk, a car ride or undertake a small errand together. Set a reasonable period of time for the activity. It is not how big or expensive an activity but that an activity was even undertaken. It is especially important if the activity acknowledges a special time or event in their life, i.e., birthday, anniversary, the death of a spouse, or the birth of a grandchild or great grandchild. The possibilities are endless. Most importantly, it is your presence that means much to them

9. **Keep the focus of talk on positive aspects of aging.** Aging is a mixed bag. The positive aspects of aging are powerful and tend to lengthen life by seven years or so. Tell positive stories, and recall positive memories. Talk of the good that is yet to come.

10. **Engage in balance exercise activities.** Balance seems to improve, at least temporarily, by engaging in muscle strengthening exercises, yoga, Tai Chi, and similar exercises. Dancing helps balance also.

## Summary

Aging is a journey indeed. It is a long journey with many unknowns and potential potholes. It is also a journey mixed with times of enjoyment and times of sadness. The journey can be facilitated by those close to us and by following a series of guidelines for the enhancement of positive and supportive relationships. By following the ten guidelines noted above, the journey can be lightened for the older persons. It will also be more enjoyable for family members and friends.

# TEN KEY FACTORS TO CONSIDER WHEN CHOOSING A RETIREMENT COMMUNITY

Selecting the right and proper retirement community is a stressful and critical decision, usually made over an extended period of time and in consultation with family members and friends. It usually is made following a trial visit, an opportunity to interview current residents of the retirement village being considered. Like many decisions in life there are several key elements that need to be explored and given careful consideration. This is particularly true when choosing a retirement community as it is most likely to be the final living community for an older individual or a couple as they face their last decade or so of life. The following ten factors are proposed as a guideline when evaluating one or more senior retirement communities.

1. **Mission Statement**
    - Why was the retirement community initially founded?
    - Under what values and belief system was it founded?
    - How are the core values and beliefs implemented and lived out within the community by the staff as well as resident life?
    - Are the core values and beliefs on paper only or are they implemented within the lifestyle of the entire community?
2. **Financial Stability**
    - Is the retirement village a non-profit or a for-profit business?
    - Is it the holding to a corporation or a group of stockholders with an underlying motive of profit?
    - How long has the retirement village been in business?
    - Is it financially supported by outside interests?
    - What kind of financial reserve are there on-hand in the event of an economic downturn? Do they have a reserve

fund that will allow them to function up to a year if there was some type of economic downturn?
- Has the retirement village been rated by Standard & Poor or Fitch's rating services? If so, what is their rating?

3. **Continuing Care**
   - Is the retirement facility a Continuing Care Retirement Community (CCRC)?
   - Do they provide multi-level care as part of the continuing care retirement community structure? That is, do they provide one, two, three, four or five levels of care?
   - Do they provide a contractual promise of access to future care and into a higher level of care as needed for any and all residents?

4. **Availability of the Continuum of Services**
   - If a multi-level service plan is available, are all services available in one location?
   - How large is the campus? Does the layout feel comfortable and are preferred services reasonably located on the campus? For example, are the rehabilitative services and the amenities located in an accessible area of the campus?

5. **Location of the Community**
   - Is the retirement community located in close proximity to a hospital, my physician's office, and other health care providers and offices?
   - Is the facility located in reasonably proximity to the cultural activities, religious services and sightseeing activities in which I may participate? Is there a shopping center nearby?
   - Is it located in close proximity to those who will visit, such as family members or friends and church members?

6. **Activities and Amenities**
   - Are there appropriate activities and amenities to meet my needs in the foreseeable future? For example, is there a swimming pool, spa, fitness center that is staffed and guided by a qualified coach?
   - Is there a full range of activities for both men and women? Is there a woodworking shop? A computer

room? Library? Access to a fax machine and other such amenities?

7. **Whole-Person Wellness**
   - Does the retirement community address the needs of the whole person including: spiritual needs, mental needs, physical needs, emotional needs and social needs?
   - Are there specific programs and ways in which these needs are met within the daily programming and activities and services available?
   - Is there a weekly chapel? Is there a chaplain? Is there a prayer room that can be used at will?

8. **The Big "What if?" Question**
   - One of the greatest fears of any one growing older is related to the possibility of their money running out before they die.
   - Does this retirement village have a plan or a way in which care will be provided even if I run out of money?
   - Are there scholarship funds and ways in which a resident who outlives his assets will be cared for and the care provided, in a respectful manner?

9. **Financial Assistance and Planning**
   - Throughout the admission process, will the retirement community administration help sell my house so the funds are available to move in?
   - Does the retirement village have assistance in the area of reviewing and modifying my will, trust, writing documents such as the durable power of attorney of healthcare and other such documents?
   - Will they assist in financial planning for the future?

10. **Financial Questions**
    - Is there a required entrance fee?
    - Is there a payment plan and various options for meeting the financial requirements?
    - What are the extra costs and extra services and how are they billed? Is there a progressive or "add-on" costs on an annual basis? What does the monthly charge include and what are all the extra costs and charges? Are they reasonable?

- Is there a possibility of a refund if circumstances change and I will need to withdraw from the facility within the first few months or year?

In reviewing the answers to the above questions, it will be easier to determine if the retirement facility is a good fit or not. It must not only feel good but be the right place at the right time with the right amenities and programs to meet the needs of which you are concerned. If so, proceed to look deeper and make the decision to go forward or not. If not, look at another facility using these same criteria. The comparison will be easier and more accurate.

Adapted from: Covenant Village, Turlock, California

# RETIRING SENIORS TAKE A BOW

Besides health, the primary concern of retiring seniors is how they want to live the rest of their lives. Secondly, they are concerned that there will be adequate funds to depend on until their death. The time to think about these concerns is long before the actual retirement time, perhaps 10-20 years so that a retirement plan and a nest egg can be generated.

The sooner the planning starts and a plan is in place, the more peace of mind will prevail and stress will lower. The lower the stress the healthier the person and the better the quality of life during the retirement years.

Research conducted by the Australian Bureau of Statistics has shown that successful aging occurs in spite of the fact that one may have one or two chronic health conditions. So, chronic illness is not a barrier to successful aging.

Here are a few suggestions to make the retirement journey go well, so you can be strong and finish well:

1. Replace the stimulation of work with social, physical, spiritual, and intellectual activities.
2. Share experiences with your spouse and family, both during the planning phase as well as living out your retirement plan.
3. Design a purpose for retirement, plan on how to live it out in daily life experiences.
4. Know that there is more to life than making money; Plan ahead for long-term financial stability by setting in place a wealth management program.

5. Develop confidence and a feeling of inner peace through financial planning, including a wealth distribution plan to occur at the time of your death.
6. Maintain a healthy lifestyle to enjoy a long-term productive life.
7. Volunteer to be of help to those in need and use it as opportunity to expand your social network.
8. Keep on meeting and getting to know new people from whom you can learn new ideas and have new experiences.
9. Consult others and attend seminars on how to make retirement the most wonderful time of your life.
10. Finish well. Plan the last few years of your life to be memorable and one that leaves a legacy of benefit for the family, community and <u>your</u> favorite charity that you wish to see supported by others after your support comes to an end.

Finally, accept the fact that we each are appointed a time to die. As any runner, such as the famous marathon runner, John Bingham knows and has said, "The finish line is out there somewhere." Until you cross that line, live fully, confidently, healthy, and productively. Share your experiences, wisdom, dreams and your personal story with others. Be social and open to new learning experiences. Draw up a personal retirement plan to cover the next 10 years. Draft it in stages if you can.

# PERSONAL LEGACY LETTER

TODAY'S DATE_____

Dear _____,

At the age of _____, I am writing this letter to you to share the personal legacy of my life. My intention is to let you know my thoughts and feelings about the life I have live, to honor the relationships that have enriched my life, and to express my gratitude to you personally. (Use extra pages as necessary)

**Reflections on my values and my life experiences:**
What I have valued most in my life is . . .
My life experience has taught me . . .

**Reflections on my cherished moments and memories:**
Some of my special memories are of . . .
I especially cherish the moments when . . .

**Reflections on my spiritual beliefs:**
What has given me strength in good and difficult times is my faith in . . .
I believe . . .

**Reflections on my desire to make amends:**
I regret the time when . . .
I wish to forgive . . .
I ask forgiveness for . . .

**Reflections on my hopes and wishes:**
My hopes for you include . . .
I ask that you consider and plan to . . .

**Reflections on my gratitude and love:**
I want to thank you for . . .
I want you to know that my love for . . .

**Reflections on my last thoughts and blessings:**
If I were saying "good-bye" to you today for the last time, I would want you to know . . .
May your life forever more be blessed with . . .

Lastly, I want to turn your attention to two meaningful prayers. I offer them to you for strength, encouragement, reflection, and purpose-driven living, so you will end well too.

## God Be With You

"God be with you 'til we meet again,
By His counsels guide uphold you,
With His peace securely fold you,
God be with you 'til we meet again

## The Irish Prayer

May the road rise to meet you.
May the wind be always at your back.
May the sun shine warm upon your face,
And the rains fall soft upon your fields.
Until we meet again,
May God hold you in the palm of His hand.

# MEMORY BUILDERS

Play your way to a renewed powerful memory. Yes, memory can be strengthened as any muscle or skill. It does take time, however. It also takes a specific set of strategies, programs, and activities to accomplish a better functioning brain, even in the older years of one's life. Here are some suggested activities in which you might choose to engage on a regular schedule to build and maintain a healthy brain.

**Change Sides.** Use your nondominant hand in activities such as tooth brushing or dialing the phone to strengthen little-used neural pathways.

**Learn to Memorize.** Four-time U.S. memory champion Scott Hagwood, who could memorize a deck of cards in two minutes flat, is an example for all of us to engage in a memory building task regularly.

**Try Do-Si-Do.** Square Dancing is known to protect against dementia, presumably because it requires multiple mental and physical skills.

**Sample the Unknown.** Card games, crossword puzzles and dominoes sharpen brain connections. For an even better cognitive workout, play with people you don't know. The randomness of the cards and dominoes and the newness of communication patterns will give your brain a vigorous workout. Novelty is like vitamins for the brain.

**Do a Mental Tune-up.** To turn a heart-healthy workout into an IQ lift, just add music, suggests a recent research study. A team at Ohio State University found that cardiac patients who exercised to music did twice as well on a test of cognitive ability compared to a group of subjects who exercised in silence. This combination of activities has been found to work well with Alzheimer's patients, as well. Exercise alone causes positive changes in the nervous system, and adding music stimulates different pathways in the brain while exercising.

**Take a Walk.** Physical exercise throughout life and especially during the older years is important to bring about maximum brain development and prevent brain weakening. With walking, the brain improves its memory functions and protects against age related brain shrinkage. Fifteen minutes of daily walking is a reasonable goal to achieve and maintain.

**Learn to Relax.** A reduction in tension in the body and mind protects against dementia. Learning to let the muscles relax, making time for meditation, and devoting time for prayer are three helpful ways to bring about a relaxed body and state of mind.

**Don't be Mad, be Glad.** The expression of positive emotions such as joy, peace, and happiness, helps the brain function more effectively than the emotional expressions of anger, sadness and depression.

**Keep on Learning.** The brain is positively stimulated by the learning of new information and skills, such as learning to play a musical instrument, learning a new language, or learning a new hobby.

**Consider the use of Medication and Supplements.** There have been many prescription medications that have come on the market over recent years. There have also been a number of new herbal supplements that may have benefit. Check with your physician regarding the options and which ones might be appropriate for you and your situation. For example, some find benefit from the use of Ginkgo Biloba, Valerian and Omega 3 Fatty Acids, to name a few.

**Eat Brain Food.** Recent research has indicated that certain foods are advantageous for use by older people. For example, broccoli, salmon, walnuts, turkey, soy beans, squash, oats, oranges, tomatoes, yogurt and blueberries are a few examples. To benefit, make all such foods part of your regular diet. And, keep the daily salt intake low, between 1,500 and 2,000 mg/day. Much of our salt intake comes from salty foods and snacks. Be careful.

# BRAIN HEALTH RELATES TO OUR BODY HEALTH

A recent Canadian research study published in *Neurology*, July 2011, underscores a link between brain health and seventeen risk factors, many of which are non-traditional and controversial. These findings are part of an ongoing series of research studies being conducted in a variety of institutions in an attempt to find a cause and affect relationship for dementia and Alzheimer's.

In this Canadian study, the researchers found that it continues to be important to be aware of and concerned for health conditions such as heart disease and diabetes, as these conditions are known to be related to the onset of dementia.

However, there were a number of less common physical conditions that appear to add a small degree of stress to the health of the brain and thereby increase the risk of dementia. These additional factors include, but are not limited to, arthritis, hearing loss, visual loss, respiratory problems, as well as stomach, bladder, and sinus problems. Stress related to feet and ankle conditions and chronic skin problems are other areas of concern. Each health condition increases the risk of dementia by approximately 3%, the researchers concluded.

The Canadian study was based on a health survey of over 7,000 Canadians 75 years of age and older who were free of dementia when the program was initiated. These people were then followed for over ten years relative to their brain functions and the onset of dementia.

*Allan G. Hedberg, Ph.D.*

For individuals without health problems initially, there was an 18% risk of developing dementia over a ten-year span. However, if one had eight health-related problems, the risk for dementia increased to about 30% over ten years. Overall, the findings also indicated that there was no particular diet or lifestyle that was effective in delaying or preventing dementia or Alzheimer's. Other studies point to the Mediterranean Diets as the proffered diet to slow down the dementia process. Further, it may not be the health factor itself but what it contributes to the lifestyle of an individual. For example, hearing loss as a secondary factor, may not create dementia itself, but it seems to contribute significantly to increased social isolation, withdrawal, and a definite reduction in overall stimulation to the brain.

The general consensus of the research indicates that a person must keep up with their general health so that they reduce the risk of dementia onset, or at least delay the onset of dementia. Other research seems to be consistently clear that the early onset of dementia or cognitive impairment results from or is related to chronic infection, excessive use of medications, chronic and untreated depression, periodontal disease, diabetes, lack of education, not engaging in sporting activities, and chronic alcohol abuse. Further, increasing age and a family history of dementia are further contributing factors to dementia. Although aging may lead to some cognitive decline, it also leads to greater insight and wisdom for better decision making.

If one were to launch an effort to delay or prevent the onset of dementia, it appears that a regular and systematic program of physical exercise is a major benefit and part of the answer. Physical exercise and an active lifestyle, and plenty of it, are to be encouraged, especially during the later years of one's life.

**HELPING YOUR BRAIN TO FUNCTION WELL**

1. Be physically active, i.e., exercise, walk, and keep moving.
2. Maintain an active social calendar, i.e., travel, attending classes, join clubs, learn a new social skill.
3. Keep your mind sharp, i.e., read, work puzzles, play music, learn a new language.
4. Quit smoking.
5. Stop drinking or greatly limit alcohol intake.
6. Manage the risk factors related to blood pressure, cholesterol, and blood glucose.
7. Maintain a positive sleep pattern of 6-8 of hours.
8. Manage body shape and weight to generally accepted levels.
9. Foster friendships and work towards increased intimacy with your loved ones.
10. Develop a faith through regular worship, studies of Holy Writ, mediation and prayer.
11. Expose yourself to 1-2 hours of sunlight or a very bright light daily.
12. Enjoy a "power nap" of one hour daily for the benefit of the brain and body.
13. Manage stress as it occurs, don't delay.
14. Manage mood states of depression, anxiety, fear and anger.

# COMING TO TERMS WITH LOSS AND GRIEF

The loss of a loved one or a significant person is an experience that almost all of us have encountered. For some of us, the loss was the moving away of a very close friend. For others, it was the wrenching experience of divorce, personal rejection or even the darkness of death. These are all examples of significant losses, but each has its own degree of emotional intensity and health related impact. We all cope differently with such losses.

Loss is considered a major experience that requires time for positive adjustment to occur. It requires understanding, emotional support, and a great deal of introspection and soul searching. Coming to terms with loss, such as a death or rejection, is facilitated by our understanding the process of grief and its resolution.

Loss generally starts with the experience of shock and denial, and eventually emerges into a state of acceptance and recovery. However, this takes time and generally follows an orderly sequence. What are the recognized stages of grief and how does one come to terms with loss?

There are five stages of grief as outlined below. Review them and see how they progress towards full recovery. This process is a very personal experience and no two people progress at the same rate or in the same manner. What follows is a general overview of the personal grief experience.

# The Journey Through The Grief Experience

### Stage one—Denial

Did it really happen? Is it really true? Numbness, feelings of shock, robot-like behavior, and acting as though nothing happened is a constant theme. Not feeling sociable or talkative is a common experience. Repressing anger, becoming isolated, and being depressed is a full time effort during this stage of grief. This stage can last days or weeks.

### Stage two—Anger

Repressing anger, dealing with self-directed anger, and the constant feeling of depression is more than anyone can handle without help. Expressing anger may feel good, but leads to strong guilty feelings. The preference is to hold anger inward. It is hard to admit to and express grief related anger.

### Stage three—Bargaining

It is common to say, "I'll do anything if you'll just bring him/her back. God, I'll change my ways, just bring him/her back." There is a reluctance to let go. Thoughts of what could have been achieved and how life could have been lived are regular and recurrent. Then there is the plea for the "magical" return of the loved one during this stage of grief.

### Stage four—Letting Go, Feeling Depressed

Increased depression is the theme. The darkness before the dawn is how a feeling is experienced. The "blah" feeling is always present. Engaging in much internal dialogue is common. Common questions include, Is this all there is to life? Why was I spared? What is my purpose now? Can I make it alone? Also, suicidal thoughts are frequent and prevailing. Discouragement is regular due to the lack of perceived progress.

Striving for personal growth; to build a new and stronger identity is the goal. Seeking a deeper purpose in living and to make life more meaningful is the constant pursuit.

**Stage five—Acceptance**

Beginning to feel free from the emotional pain of grief is now beginning to emerge. Feeling free of investing emotionally in the past relationship is also relieving. Feeling the personal progress towards greater freedom and independence is like seeing the light of day for the first time.

Although the grief process follows a fairly systematic and sequential series of steps, the one in grief often does not fully understand what is taking place at the time. Also, there is not an understanding of all the feelings within. It is even difficult to know what the normal process of grief truly is to be like.

Each of the five stages outlined above gives indication of the primary characteristics of grief at that particular stage or level. Below are a number of statements that can be checked to determine if grief is being processed and if the proper patterns of behavior are being engaged in so as to bring about appropriate and responsible recovery and calmness.

## CHECK LIST FOR MY GRIEF WORK

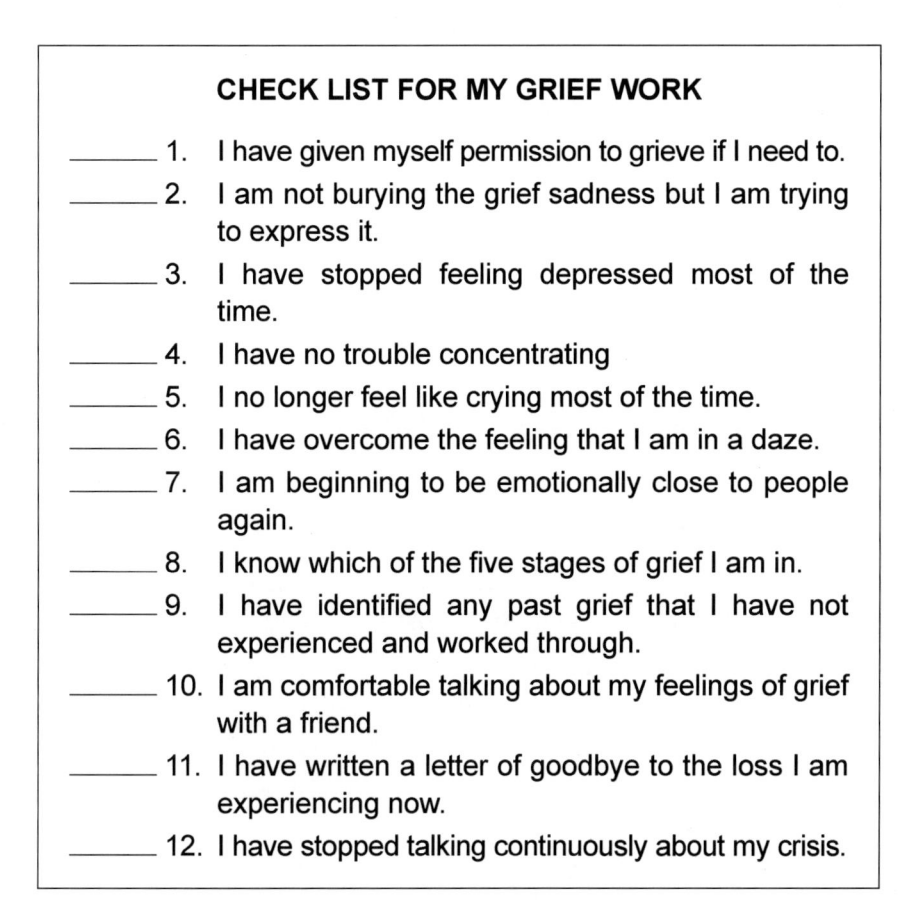

_____ 1. I have given myself permission to grieve if I need to.
_____ 2. I am not burying the grief sadness but I am trying to express it.
_____ 3. I have stopped feeling depressed most of the time.
_____ 4. I have no trouble concentrating
_____ 5. I no longer feel like crying most of the time.
_____ 6. I have overcome the feeling that I am in a daze.
_____ 7. I am beginning to be emotionally close to people again.
_____ 8. I know which of the five stages of grief I am in.
_____ 9. I have identified any past grief that I have not experienced and worked through.
_____ 10. I am comfortable talking about my feelings of grief with a friend.
_____ 11. I have written a letter of goodbye to the loss I am experiencing now.
_____ 12. I have stopped talking continuously about my crisis.

In summary, feelings of grief are the natural result of the experience of a significant loss. To lose someone through death, divorce, rejection, or by moving away is a fairly common experience for all of us. However, we all cope with loss differently. For some of us, the grief is prolonged and intense, while for others the grief is short-lived and within our abilities with which to cope. Some of us grow and mature through the loss/grief experience, while some of us become and remain bitter and resentful. Accepting the loss of a loved one is the beginning of growth. The process is a personal one. The outcome is largely determined by how we come to accept loss and our own feelings about the loss. Also, the degree in which we recover depends in part on the support system we have in place and utilized in the months following the loss event.

# Chapter Seven

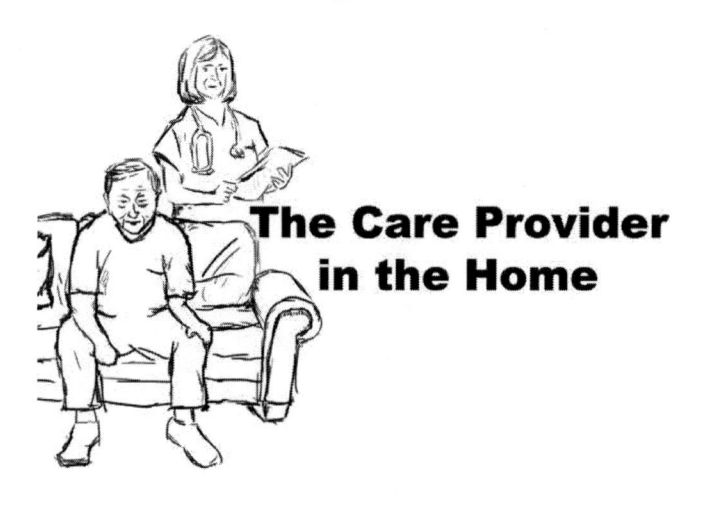

## The Care Provider in the Home

THE WORLD DOES NOT CARE WHAT YOU KNOW
UNTIL THEY KNOW THAT YOU CARE
*DAVID HARVARD*

# WORDS OF WISDOM FOR CARE PROVIDERS

To prevent burnout, the following suggestions are set forth. Add your own ideas as to how you successfully keep yourself from burnout. From the list below, note the 4 items that are most important to you (Mark with **) and the 4 items that you need to work on and do better over the next month (Mark with #).

## Guidelines for Care Providers

1. Facilitate as much independent living and self help skills as possible.
2. Spend time each week with friends as friends make good medicine; be sure to have several friends with whom you associate daily.
3. Fall-proof the home and be on guard so falls do not occur.
4. Travel now as things could change rapidly and your future chances of travel may be limited.
5. Build a "War Chest" as out of pocket costs for things and services are always greater than you planned.
6. Buy Velcro as it makes your job easier and facilitates self help.
7. Keep a journal or diary of the major happening each day as looking back on this experience may be filled with lessons to pass along to others.
8. Know the Heimlich maneuver; you may need to use it.
9. Build a provider support network as you need guidance and support as much as you give support to your loved one.
10. Educate yourself on the problems and the disease of your loved one; knowledge helps you face the "demons."

11. Lead with a positive, optimistic and hopeful attitude, but be realistic at the same time.
12. Re-shape your "box of reality;" life is not always the way you planned it or thought it was supposed to turn out.
13. Relax and enjoy the journey; don't take life too seriously.

Care providers generally accept the role of a care provider due to their emotional relationship with the impaired family member or friend. They tend to give more than they receive. Hence, burn out is very likely to occur. It usually occurs within 3 to 5 years of serving as a committed care provider.

# THE ADVANTAGES AND BENEFITS IN SERVING OLDER PEOPLE

Serving the elderly is a privilege. It is the honorable thing to do. It is the right thing to do. Serving others is an intentional act of going beyond ourselves. It is a decision to leave the safe world of our own self-centeredness and enter the world of another person to meet an identified need.

We live in a world that is self-centered, self-absorbed and narcissistic. We have been taught to look out for our self first and foremost. We have been taught to live in a self-protective and defensive mode. We have been taught the philosophy, "Get the other person first before he gets you."

Servant hood is one vocabulary word we seemed to have erased from the American dictionary. We certainly have erased it from our speaking dictionary. Yet, servant hood is what makes a person great. It makes a family great. It makes a country great. Why serve others, especially those who are in their later years of life?

## Servant Hood Makes One Great

1. **Serving gives life a new perspective.**
   The older you are the more life seems to move at a snails pace. The younger you are the more life seems to move like a rapid heart rate. A perspective of time comes from serving the elderly of our country. Perspective allows us to project what life will be like 50 years in the future. What will we accomplish in the next 50 years in comparison to what we have accomplished in the past 50 years? We ask,

"How will I contribute to the changes that will be occurring in the future." A positive perspective of others and the future promotes wonder, creative thinking and hope.

2. **Serving provides opportunity to develop special relationships.**

   Serving brings people together. Serving bonds people together. Serving allows people to become more intimate and personal with each other than otherwise would be the case. Serving allows for time to be devoted to getting to know each other, learning from each other, and growing together into a personal, deeper and meaningful relationship. Such relationships provide strength and personal well being for both the one who serves and the one who is served.

3. **Serving provides opportunity to learn about history.**

   History is learned from the textbooks, to be sure. However, the historical perspective of life through the eyes of a n older family member or close friend is priceless. Taking time to be of service to the elderly provides opportunity to sit at the feet of one who has lived and taken and lived a historical journey.

4. **Serving teaches the importance of being flexible.**

   Flexibility is a key trait of maturity and personal effectiveness. Flexibility is a key trait for all relationships to flourish. Older people are slow. They have their routines. They slowly change their mind and their moods. They often make unreasonable demands on others. All this requires flexibility in providing care and serving the elderly. As a person learns to be flexible, he/she is in a stronger position to cope with any life event and unusual life circumstances in the future.

5. **Serving puts faithfulness and persistence to a test.**

   The path of least resistance is giving up when the going gets tough. No one has ever said that serving others is a cake walk. Serving requires faithful, persistent and determined effort. Doing the right thing when no one else is paying attention is the hallmark of integrity. People of integrity faithfully and persistently serve to meet the needs of dependent elderly persons. To achieve this purpose and bring meaning to the life of the entire family, faithful and persistent service is required.

6. **Serving provides personal satisfaction in return for helping the helpless.**

   There is no greater satisfaction than to know that your efforts have made a difference in the life of someone else, particularly one who is helpless person. Feelings of satisfaction generate a corresponding sense of contentment and peace. Serving others gives a sense of empowerment and being a resource of strength for someone else. Hearing words of appreciation and gratitude is the beginning point for feelings of personal satisfaction. For a care giver, the words, "Thank you," are golden.

7. **Serving teaches the essence of compassionate care giving.**

   Life experiences teach character and skill development. Serving others, particularly the elderly is a primary life experience in which the character trait of compassion is learned. It is out of our sense of compassion for others that effective and positive care giving comes forth. As we learn to be compassionate, we are sensitive to and desire to serve the needs of others. Serving others is not just the act of giving or providing a benefit for someone else. It is, indeed, one primary way we learn about ourselves and develop new character traits as well as becoming a much better and caring person. It is through the act of serving others that we become a person of quality and a person others respect and admire.

8. **Serving prevents selfishness from being a prevailing attitude.**

   Serving other people creates a sense of caring and compassion as well as an attitude of humility. Serving others prevents selfishness from prevailing as a general attitude. It is a contradiction to provide a compassionate service for someone while at the same time being self-centered and selfish. It can't be done. Wholesome living is when we live with a sense of balance and harmony between how we behave and how we think and feel

9. **Serving allows opportunity to give back to a generation that has given much.**
   Older people know how to give. Indeed, they have given. They have given to their family, their community, their country, their churches, their clubs and organizations and to the general society. They gave without demanding a return on their investment. Serving this population is a small token of appreciation for all they have given. As one gives to someone who has given, we experience the adage, "What goes around, comes around." Tit for tat and reciprocation is an important element in all relationships. We learn this attitude in serving the elderly. We are then in a stronger position to act that way towards others in all arenas of life. Serving is an example of wholesome living.

10. **Serving symbolizes the appreciation for what senior citizens have contributed to others.**
    Older people have contributed much to their family and community. By giving of their time, they have given the best to their children, to their grandchildren, their great-grandchildren, their friends, and their country. Nothing could be a greater contribution to another individual than to share time with them. Likewise, the older people have given of themselves in wisdom in the decision-making process while guiding those younger than themselves. The older generation have given money to churches, charities, foundations and a variety of entities to provided help to the younger generation through scholarships, grants, rehabilitation services, and countless learning and personal growth experiences. Our appreciation is expressed by providing a needed service to an older person who now has a similar need as they graciously provided others in their time of need.

Indeed, serving the older generation is a learning experience and a personal growth opportunity. It can be an enjoyable investment of time and energy, with benefits for both you and the one served.

# TEENAGE VOLUNTEERS IN A SKILLED NURSING HOME

As a psychological consultant to skilled nursing facilities, I am always struck by the fact that over 60% of the patients have no visitors in the course of a year. Because of this, I have encouraged youth groups from local churches to be involved in a visitation and enrichment program for residents in the nursing facilities located near their church. This follows a similar model that churches have implemented in serving the schools located around their church by offering after school activities and reading enrichment programs.

Skilled nursing facilities serve as a training ground for students from many health care professions including physical therapy, occupational therapy, social work, speech therapy, and certified nursing assistants. Likewise, they can provide the church an opportunity for the training of junior high school and high school students in the manifestation of empathy, thoughtfulness, compassion, and Christian outreach.

Recently, while in a skilled nursing facility, I was walking down the hallway and there stood a group of seven high school students that had come to play their guitars and sing for the residents of the facility. I invited the group of teenagers into a room and encouraged them to begin singing while some visited with the three women in the room. They struck the cord of *Amazing Grace*.

While not particularly great singers, it was an emotional experience for the three patients sharing that particular room. One patient commented about how meaningful that particular hymn was to her. She began to tell the story of her life and the role the hymn, *Amazing Grace*, played in it. It should be noted that as older people listen to music, they are caused to retrieve old memories, and increase the likelihood of engaging in conversation.

One patient was so happy to see the local church group of teen singers come that he would clap and treat them to candy when they came. A close bond was formed over the months, and when he died, all the kids attended his funeral. They had lost a friend and learned a lesson on death and dying.

Research indicates that students who participate in a nursing home visitation enrichment program report positive personal experiences, such as, learning historical factual information, learning about the older generation and their lifestyle, as well as experiencing increased maturity in their own personal life.

Below is a list of needed and very practical ways in which a group of teenagers can provide a meaningful experience to residents of a nursing facility through their interaction, while gaining from it themselves.

## Music Appreciation

1. Play the piano in a central location so it is heard throughout the facility while patients are eating dinner.
2. Walk about the facility while singing, stopping at various rooms. Some sing while others visit with patients.

## Spiritual Development

1. Conduct a weekly Bible study based on specific short sections of Scripture with which the patients would be historically familiar.
2. Conduct a weekly worship service geared to the level of alertness and the spiritual level of development of the residents

3. Conduct a mid-week vesper's service with music and a brief meditation.
4. Print up and distribute a 25-word weekly devotional meditation in large print.

## Historical Perspective

1. Visit patients and engage them in conversation regarding their personal history, family history, American history, and world history.
2. Decorate billboards on historic dates such as the 4$^{th}$ of July, Memorial Day, Christmas, Thanksgiving and the anniversary and birthdays of patients.

## Computer Skills

1. Teach advanced patients basic computer skills so they can play games and e-mail family members.
2. Teach advanced computer skills to those patients that are computer literate and have families that are likewise computer literate.

## Brain Development

1. Engage students in exercises of to strengthen short-term memory.
2. Play crossword puzzles, word games, jig-saw puzzles, and board games.

## Crafts

1. Help patients with scrap booking
2. Help patients write their personal memoirs or legacy in a book or journal.

## Social Relationships

1. Sponsor birthday and anniversary recognition parties.
2. Celebrate the birthday of a famous historical figure such as Abraham Lincoln or President Eisenhower by having a party or afternoon cake time.

Youth pastors would be well-advised to make contact with several nursing homes located in the area near the church and build a relationship so that junior high and high school youth may visit the facility as volunteers on a regular and systematic basis. It is best to have weekly visits and do so in teams of six to eight students working together. The teams should be comprised of both boys and girls, some of which are older to give leadership and initiative when needed.

Before starting such a venture, it is recommended that all students undergo a dementia awareness training program. They should study the aging brain, particularly, dementia and Alzheimer's Disease. Training in how to interact socially with an older person should also be provided. Students will need to learn the protocol for appropriate behavior in a hospital. And remember, older people appreciate and value those that dress up and present themselves in a respectful and friendly manner.

Most of all, be creative and have fun. If you have fun, the residents will have fun. Always coordinate what you are going to do with the staff of the facility, usually the Recreational Therapy Department or the Social Services Department.

## A Word for the Nursing Facility Administrator

Providing a volunteer service to the residents of a nursing facility is a two way street.

The staff of the facility must be welcoming, helpful and facilitate the objectives being pursued. Setting up a schedule, providing a place to function, getting the patients up and to the location of the program being offered are just a few ways the staff can help.

Just as a church youth group leader may call and make arrangements, so can the leadership staff of the facility call and make arrangements. It is working together as a team, not just tolerating another visiting group of young do-gooders. Kids sense that they are wanted or are perceived as just being in the way. Their motivation and continuance will follow suit. Unless both parties to any volunteer service want it to happen, it will be short lived. The best action an administrator can take is to proactively appoint a staff member as the "point person" and authorize them to make it happen and do what it takes to make it a successful program.

# SELF CARE FOR CARE PROVIDERS

On an airplane, an oxygen mask descends in front of you. What do you do? As we all know, the first rule is to put on your own oxygen mask before you assist anyone else. Only when we first help ourselves can be effectively help others. Caring for yourself is one of the most fundamental, and one of the most often forgotten things you can do as a caregiver. When your needs are taken care of, the person you care for will also benefit. There are times to put yourself first, but not always, according to the Family Caregiver Alliance.

## The Risks of Care Giving

We hear often hear a wife say, "My husband is the person with Parkinson's, but now I'm the one in the hospital!" Such a situation is all too common. Researchers know a lot about the effects of caregiving on health and well-being. For example, if you are a care giving spouse between the ages of 66 and 96 and are experiencing mental or emotional strain, you are at risk for dying at a 63 percent higher rate than that of people your age who are not caregivers. The combination of loss, prolonged stress, the physical demands of caregiving, as well as the biological vulnerabilities that come with age, places the caregiver at risk for significant health problems as well as an earlier death.

Older caregivers are not the only ones who put their health and well-being at risk. If you are a baby boomer and have assumed a care giving role for parents while simultaneously juggling work and raising adolescent children, you face an increased risk for depression, chronic illness and a possible decline in quality of life.

Family care providers are also at increased risk of excessive use of alcohol, tobacco and other drugs and for depression. Studies show that an estimated 46 percent to 59 percent of caregivers are clinically depressed. Caretaking can be an emotional roller coaster. On the one hand, caring for your family member demonstrates love and commitment and can be a very rewarding personal experience. On the other hand, exhaustion, worry, inadequate resources, and continuous care demands are enormously stressful.

## Misconceptions to Correct

The following misconceptions, as identified by the Family Caregiver Alliance, need to be addressed as they in themselves cause stress and add burden.

1. I am fully responsible for my parent's health and needed care.
2. No one will do it if I don't. It is up to me.
3. If I do it right, I will get the love, attention and respect I wanted all my life.
4. I know my family thinks I never do anything right, even this effort at care giving.

Don't believe these false beliefs. Do what you can and do not try for perfection and total control. Sometimes, you can't do it good enough to please your parent or the family.

Let it go. Do what is possible and don't burn yourself out trying.

## Preventative Measures

But despite these risks, family care providers of any age are less likely than non-caregivers to practice preventive health care and self-care behavior. Regardless of age, sex, and race, and ethnicity, caregivers report problems attending to their own health and well-being while managing caregiving responsibilities. They report sleep deprivation, poor eating habits, failure to exercise, failure to stay in bed when ill, and postpone or fail to make medical and other essential appointments.

There are several measures one can undertake to prevent the burnout associated with long term care giving. The five essential steps that you, as a caregiver, must do are the following:

1. Pace yourself so you have sufficient energy throughout the day.
2. Schedule time for your own relaxation, exercise and rest.
3. Keep in regular contact with your own network of friends and support system.
4. Learn to say "no" to the excessive demands placed on you as a care giver.
5. Participate in a community support group designed for care providers and family member who assist in providing care due to the severity of a particular disorder or condition.

In summary, unless one is taking care of himself, he will have no energy or strength to help anyone. The first rule of care giving is to engage in the care taking of oneself.

# MAKING THE CARETAKING EXPERIENCE REWARDING

More than twenty-two million American households are involved in an act of caring for an ill, aged, or disabled family member. Home care is provided at a strategic time in the life of a loved one. Care giving is an intentional act where time and energy is given for the purpose of meeting the needs of a loved one. They often involve around the clock, after work and weekend duty. While the rewards of care giving are many, care givers often find themselves facing physical, emotional and financial difficulties.

Too often, care providers carryout their role of caregiving in a self-defeating and self-destructive manner. This need not be the case. Caretaking can be an experience that can be pleasant and satisfying for the caregiver as well as the care receiver. It takes teamwork to accomplish this, however. It takes a positive approach. It takes a long-term perspective.

For all care providers, there comes a time when care giving in the home needs to give way to one of the alternative care placement facilities available in the community. The following guidelines can turn the tables on a negative care taking situation and provide the caregiver with a meaningful and rewarding experience.

1. **Accept the diagnosis that has been professionally offered.** Maintain a realistic and positive expectations consistent with the future progress of the diagnosed condition. If further understanding is desired, ask the Attending Physician and professional staff.
2. **Enjoy each day with your loved one.** Enjoy each day you are able to continue to have a relationship with your loved

one. Find ways to make each day meaningful for the entire family.
3. **Maintain your own support system**. We all benefit from a support system and the cheerleaders in our life. As you provide help, and care for your loved one, maintain a relationship with the people in your life who provide you with support and encouragement. Don't go it alone.
4. **Claim peace and be anxious for nothing.** The future course of your loved one does not totally depend on you. The course of any disease or disabling condition requires the involvement of a variety of care giving resources. Utilize them cheerfully and thankfully. Ask for help, as needed.
5. **Know your own limitations.** Care giving is usually a long term commitment. Working night and day does not benefit anyone. Pace yourself. Conserve energy. Be sure you have energy needed at the end states of a disabling condition and not just during the early stages. Let others help develop a teamwork approach.
6. **Sleep well.** The extra stress and strain requires rest and a healthy sleep pattern. Remember, in the middle of the night little can be accomplished. A mid-afternoon power nap can be very beneficial. Use an alarm system in the home that provides extra security to allow for sound and restful sleep.
7. **Keep your emotions healthy**. Talk out and express your emotional feelings and experiences with those close to you. Take stress breaks, particularly when you feel the onset of irritability, agitation, and general restlessness. Confront and resolve conflicts and differences. The emotions of the care giver are just as important as the emotions of the person being cared for by the family.
8. **Think straight and concentrate**. Care giving requires positive planning and strategic thinking. There will be choice points where critical decision making is required. At such times, consult your professional and trusted resources with positive and constructive action in the best interest of all concerned.
9. **Provide healthy care by being a healthy caregiver.** It is vital that your own health be maintained. Be sure to engage

*Achieving and Living a Healthy Lifestyle in a World of Stress*

in a positive healthy living pattern so you are capable of providing the level of care needed by your loved one.

10. **Make care giving a spiritual experience**. Caring, "for the least of these," is an expressive act of faith. Caring for others gives life meaning and brings into focus the essence of life and death.

11. **Learn to delegate**. While care givers provide care on a person-to-person level, they also need to engage others in the care giving process through delegation. Ask for help. Other family members may be able to play a specific role if asked. There are many support and assistance programs available in the community. Tap all the resources available to you. You need not go it alone. There are many people and services available for specific functions or for specific and designated periods of time. They are generally available for the asking.

12. **Consult professional and non-profit organizations devoted to the particular illness or disease of your loved one.** There are a number of non-profit organizations that provide information and support that could be helpful as you provide needed care. Draw upon these resources encouragement guidance education and general information.

13. **Capitalize on the opportunity to learn lessons about family history**. Spending lengthy hours care giving also allows opportunity to discuss the history of the family and the unique experiences of various family members. This may be your best opportunity to put the family history in perspective, learn from the past and determine how you shall live in the future. Conduct interview sessions and record them on audio or video tape. Talk about the past and enjoy the events and experiences that have happened within the family.

14. **Take every opportunity to teach independent living skills and new information**. Whether your loved one is aging or disabled, they can still learn independent living skills. Information and new ideas are still worthy of being presented and taught. Assume the role of a teacher as you provide care. People are never too old to learn. Be realistic,

however. Learning something new gives encouragement and personal satisfaction. It reduces dependency.

Decisions involving the long term care of a loved one is deeply personal and emotional. A balance must be struck between the best interests of the care provider and the best interests of the one needing care. Of course, prior commitments and promises must figure in as well. Some of those early promises may have been made at a time of very different circumstances and family life considerations. An open and honest talk is the best way to resolve such dilemmas.

# FAMILY CAREGIVERS AND THEIR PRESSING CONCERNS

Approximately 65 million family members provide care for an aging or disabled family member. Of those, approximately one-half provide care for five years or longer. About a third of them provide care for more than one family member at the same time. Most of them provide assistance and daily activities greater than would be the case in a typical family relationship. It is not uncommon for such care providers to sacrifice their own quality of life and experience more personal crisis situations than typically would be the case. And, caregivers feel a great sense of burden in caring out this responsibility. The cost to American companies in lost time by the caregivers and other indirect costs is approximately $35 billion annually.

In a recent survey conducted by the National Family Caregivers Association, 1,579 family caregivers were asked a series of questions regarding the burdens they feel, the concerns they have, and the challenges they face on a daily basis as a care provider.

The findings indicate that family caregiving was considered a high burden responsibility if they assisted their loved one with personal care such as in feeding, toileting, laundry, financial management, and exercise, to name a few duties.

Further, the survey found that the caregivers with the highest level of burden included the following:

1. Those that cared for a spouse or parent who is 65 years of age or older.
2. Those that lived with the care recipient.

*Allan G. Hedberg, Ph.D.*

3. Those that felt as if they were thrown suddenly into the caregiver role as opposed to developing slowly into such a role over years.
4. Those that had been providing care for more than five years.
5. Those that cared for a loved one whose condition severely limits their ability to care for themselves such as Alzheimer's disease, Parkinson's disease, muscular dystrophy, spinal cord injury, brain injuries, and those with special care needs.

A large majority of caregivers expressed concern that they did not have enough respite care. They also expressed concerns over their own personal health, having feelings of isolation, and complained of the fact that they did not have adequate transportation for the care recipient. They also had concerns over their own financial needs and having adequate health insurance for themselves. Depression was also common among family caregivers. Up to 70% of caregivers reported depression symptoms related to care giving.

Overall, the care providers were mixed in their feelings about the level of satisfaction received in assuming this role. It was considered a thankless job. Those that personally gained from the experience did so by what they put into it and made of it. It was essentially a task of getting lemon aid from a lemon.

For help, resources and support services, see www.caregiver.org

## Chapter Eight

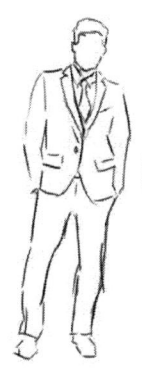

# Health Care in the Business World

DON'T FORGET UNTIL TOO LATE THAT THE BUSINESS OF
LIFE IS NOT BUSINESS, BUT LIVING
*B.C. FORBES*

# THE BENEFITS OF AN EMPLOYEE ASSISTANCE PROGRAM (EAP) FOR THE WORKER AND EMPLOYER

Employment related stress comes in many forms, unfair and unkind supervisors, competitive and jealous co-workers, and unrealistic work related time lines, to name a few. Chronic stress over time begins to have a breakdown effect on any worker. Health status is often affected among those workers exposed to chronic stress from the work place. To offer help to ill-affected employees, many companies offer an Employee Assistance Program (EAP). This program is usually offered in addition to the company's health insurance plan, but could be the primary health related benefit.

## What is an EAP?

- It is *assistance* for a troubled employee and family to maintain employability and productivity; it is not mental health therapy.
- It is *time limited*, three sessions per every six months; it is not open ended.
- It is *specific help* to diffuse a stress situation or get an employee unstuck from a problem that has been interfering with productivity and creativity; it is not the "Mr. Solve All" problem cleanser.
- It is a *confidential resource gift* for all employees and family members when tough times hit; it is not a public document or service.

*Allan G. Hedberg, Ph.D.*

## Who is the Steward of the EAP Program?

- There are many local and nationally owned EAP programs that offer the troubled employee and family member's access to local mental health providers.
- EAPs are prepared to address in a timely manner most any work related "Problem in Living." All it takes is a confidential phone call to the EAP office to locate a provider in the area in which the employee lives.
- Employment related problems are many; thirty percent are marital and family related, seven percent are health related, and twenty percent are drugs and alcohol related.
- Locally owned EAPs have the distinct advantage of immediate access to community based providers and local problem resolution should a conflict emerge.

## What are the Benefits of an EAP for the Employer?

- For those that access EAP services, quality of health increases, absenteeism reduces, employee satisfaction increases, work performance increases and the financial strength of a company is more favorable. A cost savings of $5.00 to every $1.00 invested is generally found to be the financial benefit.
- For all employees, the EAP provides wellness education and life change guidelines to prevent illness, injury, non-productivity, conflict, distraction, and absenteeism, all of which drain costs from the company's bottom line. This is one major benefit to any employer.

## Who is the Benefactor of an EAP?

- The primary benefactor is the employer and its stakeholders. The primary benefit comes from the future services of valued employees that have been saved or rehabilitated from their work stress related illness and disorders.

- The secondary benefactor is the consumer or customer of the company's product. As productivity is increased by healthy workers and costs are reduced, the products provided are made available on a more cost-equitable offering.

## What is the Benefit for the Company's HR Department?

- An opportunity to offer a new wellness product to all employees when cost savings is a primary concern to employers and employees.
- An opportunity to expand the health services a company offers employees to improve their quality of life at a small overhead cost
- An opportunity to balance the appreciated benefits between the leadership of management and labor

Be sure to check to see if your company or office has an EAP program for you and your family. If not, ask for one to be provided the employees. The cost is favorable for all concerned. Usually, a company saves more money than they spend on an EAP program and the employees get a much needed service. Indeed, a win-win situation for all.

There are also many local EAPs available to serve your company, its employees and management. Usually, the more local the vendor, the better. There are national EAP companies also that offer the same services, but managed from afar. In such situations, a personal relationship with the EAP is unlikely. When possible, stay local for your EAP service provider.

# PHYSICIAN STRESS AND ITS IMPACT ON PATIENT CARE

If you are a physician reading this article, you owe your patients a low stress life style and mind set. Your patients expect you to be managing your stress properly. A high level of chronic stress is not good for you, your profession, or your patients. If you should be feeling stressed at this time, you're not alone. 90% of physicians feel moderate to severe stress daily. But it need not be addressed alone. Share it with others to deal with it effectively.

The Estes Park Institute compiled a list of the various sources of stress contributing to the significant health related dyfunctions among practicing physicians. The findings seem very applicable to other professionals in similar situations as well. Below are the four top areas of stress for physicians. Also noted are the effects of stress and what a doctor can do to better manage stress.

As a patient of a health care provider, if you notice your doctor exhibiting stress symptoms, a kind and gentle comment might be in order. Comment that he/she looks tired, stressed or concerned. The purpose of your comment is to help a good doctor become a better doctor. Essentially, patients need to be aware of the fact that health care providers also live and work under stress. They need support as well. They are not beyond stress and its ill affects.

Consider the wide arena of doctor stress:

# I. Sources of Stress

## A. Finding Time for Everything

- How to manage office time
- How to stay on schedule yet fit in emergency patients
- How to attend meetings and find family time
- How to manage one's personal and professional lives

## B. Financial Concerns

- Pressures of increasing costs; decreasing real income
- Competition from additional physicians and managed care
- Payment issues, HMOs, malpractice, the fear of being sued
- The economy is a prime source of professional and personal stress

## C. Transitions in Medicine That Require Knowledge and Skill

- Managed care mechanisms; physician-hospital integration; group practice leadership

## D. Regulatory Issues

- Demands for peer review, OSHA coding, insurance problems, office management education, skills training, physician-hospital support services, and governmental restrictions and rules.

# II. Stress Effects on Body and Mind

## A. Effects of Stress

- Elevated blood pressure, increased blood sugar, increased heart rate, shallow and difficulty breathing
- Anxiety, anger, boredom, fatigue, frustration, moodiness, tension, self-hate and worry

- Difficulty concentrating, poor task performance, defensiveness, sleepiness, lack of focus on details, and mental blocks
- Burnout leading to conflict proneness at home and in the office/clinic

## III. Stress Management Strategies

### A. Suggested Solutions

- Work on emotional self-awareness, find time to exercise and relax
- Find professional support to help with major healthcare issues and patient skill training for better independent living.
- Learn risk management techniques to reduce rise of malpractice suits
- Seek professional counseling
- Remain calm, stay together, get enough rest and take time for your family and friends.

### B. Suggested Lifestyle Changes

- Take a mini-vacation of 3-4 days every 2-3 months
- Stop self-defeating behavior patterns such as smoking, drinking, etc.
- Lower personality style from Type A to Type B.

Overall, stress not only impacts and impairs a doctor's health, but it can also impair his performance and exercise of skill. It also impairs relationships in the office, relationships with colleagues and with his patients. Anger management training will improve energy levels, interpersonal skills, and mood. One cannot afford to let stress go unaddressed or ignored. The price is too great for all parties. Don't call stress by another name and try and fool yourself either. It is what it is. Be honest and do what is necessary to keep yourself fit and maintain a low stress working condition and office environment.

To be sure, high and chronic stress leads to mistakes and errors in treatment, record keeping and being timely in responding to requests of patients and regulatory agencies. High stress can also lead to very inappropriate behavior, such as, drug use, alcohol use, absenteeism, sickness and a grouchy disposition, to name a few. Overall, stress in the office and in the life of the health care worker will impact the doctor/patient relationship and the doctor/staff relationship.

# NEGOTIATING WITH YOUR HEALTH CARE PROVIDER

Would you be surprised to learn that only a small portion of patients pay 100% of the bill they receive from their health care provider for services rendered? This includes hospitals, clinics, labs, and specialists. It is not uncommon for a 10-30% discount to be arranged for lowering the final billing statement. Others commonly work out payment plans with a portion of the final billing being forgiven.

It is important to be aware of the fact that health care providers and medical facilities commonly have a rate schedule that is utilized differently for different patients. Some are offered a lower rate, others pay a percentage. Offering a fluctuation in the billing rate is not uncommon for most health care providers. Patients might be encouraged to consider negotiating with their health care provider for an acceptable rate prior to the rendering of any particular service. Hence, negotiating may not only be a smart thing to do but it might be a prudent thing to do given your own financial circumstances and today's economy.

Remember, negotiations are not only permissible with physicians but also include physical therapists, psychologists, speech therapists, chiropractors, dentists, social workers, marriage and family counselors, and other types of health care providers. Remember that your health care provider must set fees and charge consistent with the ethics of their profession and in fairness to other patients. Negotiations can only go so far. Be realistic in your expectations.

Below are a few suggested negotiating tips that might be utilized with your health care provider as you anticipate services being rendered to you in the future. Fees and payment plans might be negotiated each time a procedure is being undertaken, or as a general agreement that you establish with your health care provider for all services rendered in the future.

## Negotiating Tips

1. **With humility and respect, speak up assertively.** Effective communication is assertive communication. Your doctor is accustomed to dealing with patients who speak up assertively but demonstrate respect in what they say and how it is expressed. If you are going to negotiate, first determine the desired outcome and then request it assertively.
2. **Request a discount in fees upon your willingness to pay cash at the time services are rendered.** Before making such a request, determine what discount percentage you would like to request and be prepared to pay when services are rendered. You must follow through on such a request if the doctor agrees to it.
3. **Ask if the sessions can be sub-divided into smaller segments of time for a lower rate.** There are times when the cost could be lower if the sessions were divided over time. If you are only able to pay a certain amount, then ask the doctor to restrict or pace services rendered in keeping with that amount.
4. **Ask if the treatment sessions can be spread out over a period of time so that payment is not burdensome in any given month.** Spreading out a diagnostic and treatment plan could be helpful so that payment keeps pace with services rendered. For example, perhaps lab work could be spread out over a period of time rather than having it all done at once which may require a higher total payment when you can least afford it.
5. **Be honest and request special arrangements only if you really need it.** Be honest and clear with your doctor if you make any special requests of the doctor to provide you a service in a particular way or in a particular format. Likewise, be sure that any special requests for diagnostic testing or

procedures are absolutely necessary. If not, do not agree to such procedures or tests or delay them until you can pay for them. The doctor will understand.

6. **Request a payment plan over the course of 12 months and intend to have it paid off by then.** A payment plan over a period of time such as 12 months is not uncommon. It is reasonable to ask for it but it must be done with the full intent that payments will be made faithfully and in a timely manner.

7. **Ask for samples of medication and other medical supplies.** Doctors get samples from the sales representatives and are able to make those available to their patients on an as-needed basis. If you need a particular medical supply or medication, do not hesitate to ask if samples are available that could be obtained for your use. Samples could help you not only try the medication but reduce your costs for at least a few weeks or a month or so. If the samples are not helpful, you may not want to purchase a full prescription that is costly and may be a waste of your money. If in doubt, request samples.

8. **Ask for all medications to be prescribed at the lowest cost such as use of generics or an equivalent medication that might cost less than the preferred medication.** Most medications are available in the generic form at less cost. Be sure that you indicate to your doctor that you are willing to take medication in a generic form to save costs. While some doctors do this routinely, yours may not do so but would if you requested it.

9. **Ask to see a Physician Assistant, or other allied professional if the charges are less than those charged by the doctor.** Most doctors have allied staff members in their offices such as a physician assistant. Often the billing rate to see an allied professional is less than the doctor's rate. Consider when you make an appointment if your situation could be handled by the physician assistant and only see the doctor if absolutely necessary. Ask if this is reasonable when making your appointment.

10. **Consider paying with your credit card to rack up mileage points for your next air flight.** If you travel or use your credit card for secondary benefits such as airline mileage, be sure to pay with credit cards. While this costs the doctor a few small percentage points, it could be a great help to you.

Negotiating is not to get some type of great deal, but a fair deal for all. It must be a Win-Win outcome to be a fair deal. Be honest and speak with integrity. Remember, your future doctor/patient relationship needs to be maintained and strengthened by any such discussions.

# WHEN DEPRESSION COMES TO THE WORK PLACE

You cannot define it but you know it when it hits. Deep within the Black Hills in South Dakota is the famous 100 mile long Wind Cave. Touring the Wind Cave, you come to a point along the tour at which time the tour guide gathers everybody close together and then turns off the electric lights lining the cave. Immediately, a thick darkness prevails and engulfs you. In an instant, you experience all the emotions commonly associated with a pale of depression. You become frightened, disoriented, helpless, paralyzed, choked up, and feeling very much alone.

While depression has been part of the human experience since the beginning of time, it was incorporated into the language of the professional community when Hippocrates referred to it 2500 years ago as melancholia. Today, we not only recognize it and have a better understanding of it, but we also have a fairly good grasp on how to prevent it and how to treat it. Still, it remains the "disease of the decade."

Depression deeply impacts marital relationships, parent-child relationships, our friendship circle, and our colleague relationships that provide strength, encouragement and support. Likewise, depression impairs every component of an employee's work performance. It interferes with the ability to produce a timely, accurate, creative, and well-conceived work product.

## CONSIDER THE FACTS:

Clinical depression has become one of America's most costly illnesses. It ranks among the top 3 work place problems. 3% of total short-term disability days are due to depressive disorders. If left untreated, the cost to the U.S. economy is approximately $45 billion dollars annually in absenteeism, lost productivity, and direct treatment costs. That is approximately $600.00 per depressed worker per year. Over 200 million work days are lost each year due to depression. A study by the Rand Corporation found that depressed patients spend more days in bed than those with diabetes, arthritis, back problems, lung problems, or gastrointestinal disorders. When alcoholism and drug abuse is involved, costs escalate and work performance further depreciates. Depression saps the most precious skills a worker brings to the work place—concentration, decision making, judgment, creativity, energy, and concentration, to name a few. The age group most vulnerable to depression is those in the prime working years, age 24 to 44.

## WHAT MANAGERS NEED TO KNOW

* If an employee becomes imperiled by depression, immediately take constructive and restorative action guided by the American Disabilities Act. Time off, flex time, light duty, change of assignment, change of supervisors, reduced time, modifications in work expectations, and assigning a mentor are just of the few options to be considered. It is a goal to keep an employee productive, yet be supported and assisted in overcoming the dark enemy that can rob the work place of a valued employee.
* Help the impaired employee draw upon a network of professionals who can assist along the path of recovery to full and productive employment. Be sure the EAP program is utilized. Be sure the mental health insurance plan is fully utilized. Help the employee connect with a local therapist with whom there has been a working relationship or professional respect and confidence.

* Support the impaired employee and his or her family in the journey of recovery. Call the spouse. Encourage the family. Offer needed assistance. Be willing to personally visit the employee at critical points in his or her journey of recovery.
* Develop a plan for return to employment. Set guidelines. Provide stepping stones. Make it easy to come back and resume one's responsibilities, even if it is undertaken in steps from light duty to full duty, from part-time to full-time employment.
* Annually review corporate medical, mental health, and EAP programs and benefits. Make sure HR and the EAP representative are trained to make appropriate referrals and provide needed assistance consistent with policies and practices. And, educate employees by reproducing and distributing brochures, pamphlets, and relevant websites. Consider developing a corporate mental health and stress management policy.

## WHAT DEPRESSED EMPLOYEES NEEDS TO KNOW

* Correct irrational thinking. For example, not all projects and ideas proposed need be approved by management. Further, it is not necessary to be thoroughly competent, adequate, and achieving in all respects of work. It is perfectly acceptable to seek consultation and gather ideas from a variety of sources rather than being the sole source of a proposed plan or idea.
* Learn to be self-complimentary. When you know you have done a good job or performed well, pause and reflect on a complimentary phrase about your performance and yourself. Do not be totally dependent upon management and colleagues to compliment you and your performance. While management should be generous in providing complimentary feedback to employees, some managers do not ascribe to such a principle or were not raised in a home in which compliments and affirmation were not daily verbal expressions. If a manager or colleague did not learn

to affirm others, he or she will not affirm you, even when you think you deserve it.
* Seek time with colleagues who are encouraging and are positive in their attitudes and speech. In every work environment, there are people who are encouragers and those who are discouragers. There are those who support and those who depreciate others. Avoid the negative people, or help them change. The prevailing attitude of the work force strongly affects the performance and productivity of a company. The emotional tone of the work place affects every worker's level of creativity, accuracy, and output as well as their emotional health. A healthy work environment is characterized by general happiness, mutual respect and appreciation for colleagues, and agreement with the purpose and mission for which a company is in business.
* You have the right to assertive communication patterns. Rather than being passive and absorb unwanted and unpleasant communications from others, it is essential that you express your feelings, desires, needs, and preferences. There are times to say "no" and times to say "yes." There are times to ask for help. Learn to get from others what you need and want. Control the degree to which other people overpower or try to control you. Engage in assertive communication so others can better understand you and respond to your needs in a more satisfying manner. Speak up and stop undesirable and unwanted behavior patterns, gestures, verbal expressions, and other innuendoes that create feelings of depression, anxiety, and distress.
* When faced with a major problem or burdensome task, undertake the problem solving process one step at a time. Be success oriented. Identify the steps that need to be undertaken to accomplish the task. Start from the known and proceed to the unknown. Start with the simple steps and proceed to the more complex steps. Seek out and accept help from colleagues and management, as needed. Remember, you are not alone. There are others who are willing and able to join in with you so success and accomplishment is achieved in a timely manner.

*Allan G. Hedberg, Ph.D.*

## WHAT WE ALL NEED TO KNOW

Success in the work place depends on everyone's contribution. No one can afford to ignore the early signs of depression. It affects approximately 10% of the population. The good news is that, in more than 80% of cases, treatment is effective. The combination of psychotherapy and appropriate antidepressant medication has been demonstrated to be the most effective treatment plan to help a depressed person return to a satisfactory functioning life at home and in the work place. It is not a matter of coping with depression, but changing it by changing lifestyle, circumstances, and behavioral patterns.

Published in *Valley Health Magazine*, May/June, 2007

# EPIGRAPH

### TAKE TIME TO THINK AND BE HEALTHY

Take time to think; it is the source of creative ideas.
Take time to play; it is the secret of perpetual youth.
Take time to read; it is the fountain of wisdom.
Take time to laugh; it is the music of the soul.
Take time to give; it is the way to warm the heart.
Take time to express thanks; it is the road to happiness.
Take time to help others; it is a blessing to them and you.
Take time to pray; it is letting go and letting God have his way.
Take time to be healthy, it is the way to live on a higher plane.

Author Unknown

ACHIEVING AND LIVING A HEALTHY LIFESTYLE
IN A WORLD OF STRESS
Allan G. Hedberg, Ph.D.
Shaw Sixth Square
5100 N. Sixth St.140
Fresno, CA 93710
allanghedberg@sbcglobal.net
Phone 559-244-3260
Fax 559 227 6149

The book may be ordered online from www.Authorhouse.com.